Gastrointestinal Physiology

Fifth Edition

Edited by

Leonard R. Johnson, PhD

Thomas A. Gerwin Professor and Chairman
Department of Physiology and Biophysics
University of Tennessee Health Sciences Center
Memphis, Tennessee

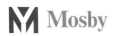 Mosby

St. Louis Baltimore Boston Carlsbad Chicago Naples New York Philadelphia Portland
London Madrid Mexico City Singapore Sydney Tokyo Toronto Wiesbaden

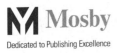
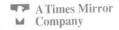

Mosby

Dedicated to Publishing Excellence

A Times Mirror Company

Vice President and Publisher: Anne S. Patterson
Editor: Emma D. Underdown
Developmental Editor: Christy Wells
Project Manager: Linda Clarke
Associate Production Editor: Kathleen E. Hillock
Series Designer: Elizabeth Fett
Manufacturing Manager: William A. Winneberger, Jr.
Cover Art: G. W. Graphics

Printed in the United States of America
Composition by Top Graphics
Printing/binding by R.R. Donnelley & Sons Co.

Mosby-Year Book, Inc.
11830 Westline Industrial Drive
St. Louis, Missouri 63146

Library of Congress Cataloging in Publication Data

Gastrointestinal physiology /√edited by Leonard R. Johnson. — 5th ed.
    p.   cm.
    Includes bibliographical references and index.
    ISBN 0-8151-4934-4
    1. Gastrointestinal system—Physiology.   2. Digestion.
I. Johnson, Leonard R.
    [DNLM: 1. Gastrointestinal System—physiology. WI 102 G2571
1997]
QP145.G27 1997
612.3—dc20
DNLM/DLC
for Library of Congress   96-30466
                                     CIP

97 98 99 00 01 / 9 8 7 6 5 4 3 2 1

Contributors

Eugene D. Jacobson, MD
Professor, Departments of Internal Medicine
and Physiology
University of Colorado Health Sciences Center
Denver, Colorado

Leonard R. Johnson, PhD
Thomas A. Gerwin Professor and Chairman
Department of Physiology and Biophysics
University of Tennessee Health Sciences
Center
Memphis, Tennessee

Norman W. Weisbrodt, PhD
Professor, Department of Integrative Biology
University of Texas Medical School
Houston, Texas

Preface

The first edition of *Gastrointestinal Physiology* appeared in 1977. It developed as a result of the authors' teaching experiences and need for a book on gastrointestinal physiology written and designed for medical students and beginning graduate students. This fifth edition is written by the same authors and directed to the same audience. As with any new edition, those involved believe that it is significantly better than the previous one. The contributors and I feel strongly that this edition is such an improvement. All chapters contain significant amounts of new material and have been brought up-to-date with current information—without introducing undue amounts of controversy to confuse students.

The fifth edition has two added features that we feel will assist students in understanding the material. First, key words now appear in bold type the first time they are defined. Second, a summary of the major concepts is included at the end of each chapter. This is meant to aid the student in organizing his or her thoughts about the material presented.

The entire book is still written by the original authors. I am again indebted to them for their ability to transmit their expertise in a lucid and concise manner. Their contributions arrived on schedule, and anyone who has had the experience of editing a volume realizes how rare it is.

We are all grateful to our own students for pointing out ways to improve the book. Numerous colleagues in other medical schools and professional institutions have added their suggestions and criticisms as well. We are thankful for their interest and help, and we hope that anyone having criticisms of this edition or suggestions for improving future editions will transmit them to us.

Finally, I thank Ms. Easter Jenkins for typing my own chapters and helping with the communications and organizational work that are a necessary part of such a project.

Leonard R. Johnson

Contents

Regulation

Peptides of the Gastrointestinal Tract

Leonard R. Johnson

The functions of the gastrointestinal (GI) tract are regulated by peptides, derivatives of amino acids, and a variety of mediators released from nerves. All GI hormones are peptides. It is important, however, to realize that not all peptides found in digestive tract mucosa are hormones. The GI tract peptides can be divided into endocrines, paracrines, and neurocrines, depending on the method by which the peptide is delivered to its target site.

Endocrines or hormones are released into the general circulation and reach all tissues (unless excluded from the brain by the blood-brain barrier). Specificity is a property of the target tissue itself. Specific receptors, which recognize and bind the hormone, are present on its target tissues and absent from others. There are four established GI hormones; in addition, some GI peptides are released from endocrine cells into the blood but have no known physiologic function. Conversely, several peptides have been isolated from mucosal tissue and have potent GI effects, but no mechanism for their physiologic release has been found. Members of these latter two groups are classified as candidate hormones.

Paracrines are released from endocrine cells and diffuse through the extracellular space to their target tissues. Their effects are limited by the short distances necessary for diffusion. Nevertheless, these agents can affect large areas of the digestive tract by virtue of the scattered and abundant distributions of the cells containing them. A paracrine agent also can act on endocrine cells. Thus a paracrine may release or inhibit the release of an endocrine substance, thereby ultimately regulating a process remote from its origin. Histamine, a derivative of the amino acid histidine, is an important regulatory agent that acts as a paracrine.

Some GI peptides are located in nerves and may act as **neurocrines** or neurotransmitters. A neurocrine is released near its target tissue and needs only to diffuse across a short synaptic gap. Neurocrines conceivably may stimulate or inhibit the release of endocrines or paracrines. **Acetylcholine** (ACh), although not a peptide, is an important neuroregulator in the GI tract. One of its actions is to stimulate acid secretion from the gastric parietal cells.

■ GENERAL CHARACTERISTICS

The GI tract is the largest endocrine organ in the body. Its hormones were the first to be discovered. The word "hormone" was coined by W. B.

Hardy and used by Starling in 1905 to describe secretin and gastrin and to convey the concept of bloodborne chemical messengers. The GI hormones are released from the mucosa of the stomach and small intestine by nervous activity, distention, and chemical stimulation coincident with the intake of food. Released into the portal circulation the GI hormones pass through the liver to the heart and back to the digestive system to regulate its movements and secretions. These hormones also regulate the growth of the stomach, small intestine, and pancreas.

The GI peptides have many different types of actions. Their effects on water, electrolyte, and enzyme secretion are well known; but they also influence motility, growth, and the release of other hormones, as well as intestinal absorption. Many of these actions overlap; two or more GI peptides may affect the same process in the same direction, or they may inhibit each other. Many of the demonstrated actions of these peptides are pharmacologic and do not occur under normal circumstances. This chapter is concerned primarily with the physiologic effects of the GI peptides.

The actions of the GI peptides also may vary in both degree and direction among species. The actions discussed in the remainder of this chapter are those occurring in humans.

■ DISCOVERY

Four steps are required to establish the existence of a GI hormone. First, a physiologic event such as a meal must be demonstrated to provide the stimulus to one part of the digestive tract that subsequently alters the activity in another part. Second, the effect must persist after all nervous connections between the two parts of the tract have been severed. Third, from the site of application of the stimulus a substance must be isolated that, when injected into the blood, mimics the effect of the stimulus. Fourth, the substance must be identified chemically and its structure confirmed by synthesis.

Five GI peptides have achieved full status as hormones. They are secretin, gastrin, cholecystokinin (CCK), gastric inhibitory peptide (GIP), and motilin.

There is an extensive list of "candidate" hormones, whose significance has not been established. This list includes several chemically defined peptides that have significant actions in physiology or pathology but whose hormonal status has not been proved. These are pancreatic polypeptide, neurotensin, and substance P. In addition, two known hormones, glucagon and somatostatin, have been identified in GI tract mucosa. Their possible function as GI hormones is currently being investigated. Some of these peptides function physiologically as paracrines or neurocrines.

Secretin, the first hormone, was discovered in 1902 by Bayliss and Starling and was described as a substance, released from the duodenal mucosa by hydrochloric acid, that stimulated pancreatic bicarbonate and fluid secretion. It was isolated and its amino acid sequence was identified by Jorpes and Mutt in 1966. It was synthesized by Bodanszky and co-workers later in the same year.

Edkins discovered **gastrin** in 1905, stating to the Royal Society that "in the process of the absorption of digested food in the stomach a substance may be separated from the cells of the mucous membrane which, passing into the blood or lymph, later stimulates the secretory cells of the stomach to functional activity." For 43 years investigators were preoccupied by the controversy over the existence of gastrin. The debate intensified when Popielski demonstrated that histamine, a ubiquitous substance present in large quantities throughout the body (including the gastric mucosa), was a powerful gastric secretagogue. In 1938 Komarov demonstrated that gastrin was a polypeptide and was different from histamine. By 1964 Gregory and his colleagues had extracted and isolated hog gastrin. It was synthesized by Kenner and his group in the same year. After 60 years all of the criteria for establishing the existence of a GI hormone had been satisfied.

In 1928 Ivy and Oldberg described a humoral mechanism for the stimulation of gallbladder contraction initiated by the presence of fat in the intestine. The hormone was named **cholecystokinin** after its primary action. The only controversy involving cholecystokinin is a mild one over nomenclature. In 1943 Harper and Raper described a hormone released from the small intestine that stimulated pancreatic enzyme secretion and accordingly named it pancreozymin. As the purification of these two substances was carried out by Jorpes and Mutt in 1968, it became obvious that both properties resided in the same peptide. For the sake of convenience and because it was the first action described, this hormone was called cholecystokinin.

In 1969 Brown and his co-workers described the purification of a powerful enterogastrone from intestinal mucosa. **Enterogastrone** literally means substance from the intestine (*entero-*) that inhibits (*-one*) the stomach (*gastr-*). By 1971 this peptide had been purified, isolated, sequenced, and named **gastric inhibitory peptide** after its ability to inhibit gastric secretion. Released from the intestinal mucosa by fat and glucose, GIP also stimulates insulin release. Following the proof that release of insulin was a physiologic action of the peptide, GIP became the fourth GI hormone. The insulinotropic effect of GIP requires elevated amounts of serum glucose. For this reason, and because it is doubtful whether the inhibitory effects of the peptide on the stomach are physiologic, it has been suggested that its name be changed to (G)lucose-dependent (I)nsulinotropic (P)eptide. In either case it is still referred to as GIP.

Brown and his co-workers also described the purification of **motilin** in the early 1970s. Motilin is a linear 22–amino acid peptide purified from the upper small intestine. During fasting it is released cyclically and stimulates upper gastrointestinal motility. Its release is under neural control and accounts for the interdigestive migrating myoelectric complex.

■ **CHEMISTRY**

The GI hormones and some related peptides can be divided into two structurally homologous families.

The first consists of gastrin (Figure 1-1) and CCK (Figure 1-2). The five carboxy-terminal (C-terminal) amino acids are identical in these two hormones. All the biologic activity of gastrin can be reproduced by the four C-terminal amino acids. This tetrapeptide, then, is the minimal

1	2	3	4	5	6-10	11
Pyro —	Gly —	Pro —	Trp —	Leu —	(Glu)5 —	Ala —

12	13	14	15	16	17
Tyr —	Gly ┬	Trp —	Met —	Asp —	Phe — NH₂

Tyr
|
R   Minimal fragment for strong activity

Gastrin I, R = H   Pyropyroglutamyl
Gastrin II, R = SO₃H

Figure 1-1 ■ Structure of human little gastrin (G 17).

1	2	3	4	5	6	7	8	9
Lys —	Ala —	Pro —	Ser —	Gly —	Arg —	Val —	Ser —	Met —

10	11	12	13	14	15	16	17	18
Ile —	Lys —	Asn —	Leu —	Gln —	Ser —	Leu —	Asp —	Pro —

19	20	21	22	23	24	25	26
Ser —	His —	Arg —	Ile —	Ser —	Asp —	Arg —	Asp —

27	28	29	30	31	32	33
Tyr —	Met ┬	Gly —	Trp —	Met —	Asp —	Phe — NH₂

SO₃H   Identical to gastrin

Minimal fragment for CCK pattern of activity

Figure 1-2 ■ Porcine CCK.

fragment of gastrin needed for strong activity and is about one-sixth as active as the whole 17–amino acid molecule. The sixth amino acid from the C-terminus of gastrin is tyrosine, which may or may not be sulfated. When sulfated, the hormone is called **gastrin II.** Both forms occur with equal frequency in nature. The N-terminus of gastrin is pyroglutamyl, and the C-terminus is phenylalamide (Figure 1-1). Note that the NH_2 group following Phe does not signify that this is the N-terminus but that this C-terminal amino acid is amidated. These alterations in structure protect the molecule from aminopeptidases and carboxypeptidases.

CCK, which has 33 amino acids, contains a sulfated tyrosyl residue in position 7 from the C-terminus. CCK can activate gastrin receptors (e.g., those for acid secretion, also called CCK-B receptors); gastrin can activate CCK receptors (e.g., those for gallbladder contraction, also called CCK-A receptors). Each hormone, however, is much more potent at its own receptors than at those of its homologue. CCK is always sulfated in nature, and desulfation produces a peptide with the gastrin pattern of activity. The minimally active fragment for the CCK pattern of activity is

therefore the C-terminal heptapeptide. In summary, peptides belonging to the gastrin-CCK family having a tyrosyl residue in position 6 from the C-terminus or in position 7 and unsulfated possess the gastrin pattern of activity—strong stimulation of gastric acid secretion and weak contraction of the gallbladder. Peptides with a sulfated tyrosyl residue in position 7 have cholecystokinetic potency and are weak stimulators of gastric acid secretion. Obviously the tetrapeptide itself and all fragments less than seven amino acids long possess gastrin-like activity.

The second group of peptides is homologous to secretin and includes **vasoactive intestinal peptide** (VIP), GIP, and **glucagon** in addition to secretin (Figure 1-3). Secretin has 27 amino acids, all of which are required for substantial activity. Pancreatic glucagon has 29 amino acids, 14 of which are identical to those of secretin. Glucagon-like immunoreactivity has been isolated from the small intestine, but the significance of this **enteroglucagon** has not been established. Glucagon has no active fragment, and like secretin the whole molecule is required before any activity is observed. There is evidence that secretin exists as a helix; thus the entire

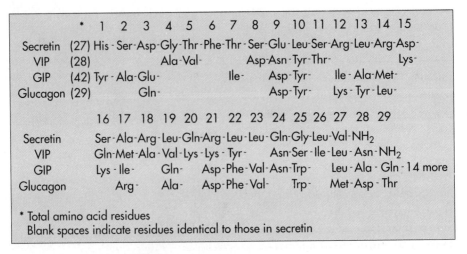

	*	1	2	3	4	5	6	7	8	9	10	11	12	13	14	15
Secretin	(27)	His-	Ser-	Asp-	Gly-	Thr-	Phe-	Thr-	Ser-	Glu-	Leu-	Ser-	Arg-	Leu-	Arg-	Asp-
VIP	(28)			Ala-	Val-				Asp-	Asn-	Tyr-	Thr-				Lys-
GIP	(42)	Tyr-	Ala-	Glu-				Ile-		Asp-	Tyr-		Ile-	Ala-	Met-	
Glucagon	(29)			Gln-						Asp-	Tyr-		Lys-	Tyr-	Leu-	

	16	17	18	19	20	21	22	23	24	25	26	27	28	29
Secretin	Ser-	Ala-	Arg-	Leu-	Gln-	Arg-	Leu-	Leu-	Gln-	Gly-	Leu-	Val-	NH_2	
VIP	Gln-	Met-	Ala-	Val-	Lys-	Lys-	Tyr-		Asn-	Ser-	Ile-	Leu-	Asn-	NH_2
GIP	Lys-	Ile-		Gln-		Asp-	Phe-	Val-	Asn-	Trp-		Leu-	Ala-	Gln - 14 more
Glucagon		Arg-		Ala-		Asp-	Phe-	Val-		Trp-		Met-	Asp-	Thr

* Total amino acid residues
  Blank spaces indicate residues identical to those in secretin

Figure 1-3 ■ Structures of secretin family of peptides.

amino acid sequence may be necessary to form a tertiary structure with biologic activity.

GIP and VIP each have nine amino acids that are identical to those of secretin. Each has many of the same actions as secretin and glucagon. This group of peptides will be discussed in greater detail later in the chapter.

Most peptide hormones are heterogeneous and occur in two or more molecular forms. Gastrin, secretin, and CCK have all been shown to exist in more than one form. Gastrin was originally isolated from hog antral mucosa as a heptadecapeptide (Figure 1-1), which is now referred to as **little gastrin or G 17.** It accounts for 90% of antral gastrin. Yalow and Berson demonstrated heterogeneity by showing that the major component of gastrin immunoactivity in the serum was a larger molecule that they called **big gastrin.** On isolation big gastrin was found to contain 34 amino acids; hence it is called **G 34.** Trypsin splits G 34 to yield G 17 plus a heptadecapeptide different from G 17. Therefore G 34 is not simply a dimer of G 17. An additional gastrin molecule (G 14) has been isolated from tissue and contains the C-terminal tetradecapeptide of gastrin. Current evidence indicates that most G 17 is produced from pro G 17 and most G 34 from pro G 34. Thus G 34 is not a necessary intermediate in the production of G 17.

During the interdigestive (basal) state most human serum gastrin is G 34. Unlike that of other species, the duodenal mucosa of humans contains significant amounts of gastrin. This is primarily G 34 and is released in small amounts during the basal state. After a meal a large quantity of antral gastrin, which is primarily G 17, is released and provides most of the stimulus for gastric acid secretion. Smaller amounts of G 34 are released from both the antral and the duodenal mucosa. G 17 and G 34 are equipotent, although the half-life of G 34 is 38 minutes and that of G 17 is about 7 minutes.

■ DISTRIBUTION AND RELEASE

The GI hormones are located in endocrine cells scattered throughout the GI mucosa from the stomach through the colon. The cells containing individual hormones are not clumped together but are dispersed among the epithelial cells. The nature of this distribution makes it virtually impossible to surgically remove the source of one of the GI hormones and examine the effect of its absence without compromising the digestive function of the animal.

The endocrine cells of the gut are members of a widely distributed system termed **amine precursor uptake decarboxylation** (APUD) cells. These cells are all derived from neuroendocrine-programmed cells originating in the embryonic ectoblast.

The distributions of the individual gastrointestinal hormones are shown in Figure 1-4. Gastrin is most abundant in antral and duodenal mucosa.

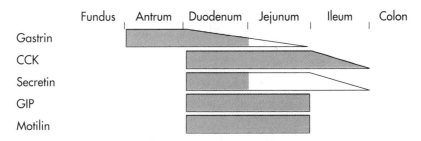

Figure 1-4 ■ Distribution of the GI hormones. Shaded areas indicate where most release occurs under normal conditions.

Most of its release under physiologic conditions is from the antrum. Secretin, CCK, GIP, and motilin are found in the duodenum and jejunum.

Ultrastructurally, GI endocrine cells have hormone-containing granules concentrated at their bases close to the capillaries. The granules discharge, releasing their hormones in response to a number of events that are either the direct or the indirect result of neural, physical, and chemical stimuli associated with eating a meal and the presence of that meal within the digestive tract. These endocrine cells have microvilli on their apical borders that presumably contain receptors for sampling the luminal contents.

Table 1-1 lists the stimuli that are physiologically important releasers of the GI hormones. Gastrin and motilin are the only hormones demonstrated to be released directly by neural stimulation. Protein in the form of peptides and single amino acids releases both gastrin and CCK. Fatty acids containing eight or more carbon atoms or their monoglycerides are the most potent stimuli for CCK release. That fat must be broken down into an absorbable form before releasing CCK is evidence that the receptors for release are triggered during the process of absorption. Carbohydrate, the remaining major food-

stuff, does not alter the release of gastrin, secretin, or CCK but does stimulate GIP release. GIP also is released by fat and protein. The strongest stimulus for secretin release is hydrogen ion. Secretin is released when the pH in the duodenum falls below 4.5. Secretin also is released by fatty acids. This may be a significant mechanism for secretin release because the concentration of fatty acids in the lumen is often high. CCK also can be released by acid, but, except during hypersecretion of acid, the physiologic significance of this mechanism of release has not been established. The purely physical stimulus of distention activates antral receptors, causing gastrin release; for example, inflating a balloon in the antrum will release gastrin. During a meal the pressure of ingested food initiates this response. The magnitude of the response is not as great as originally believed, however, and the contribution that distention makes to the total amount of gastrin released in humans is probably minor. Gastrin also can be released by calcium, decaffeinated coffee, and wine. Pure alcohol in the same concentration as the alcohol in wine does not release gastrin but does stimulate acid secretion. Motilin is released cyclically (approximately every 90 minutes) during fasting.

TABLE 1-1

Releasers of gastrointestinal hormones

	Hormones				
	Gastrin	CCK	Secretin	GIP	Motilin
Protein	S	S	O	S	O
Fat	O	S	S–	S	S–
Carbohydrate	O	O	O	S	O
Acid	I	S–	S	O	S–
Distention	S	O	O	O	O
Nerve	S	O	O	O	S

S, Physiologic stimulus for release; S–, of secondary importance; O, no effect; I, inhibits release physiologically.

This release is prevented by atropine and the ingestion of a mixed meal. Acid and fat in the duodenum, however, increase motilin release.

In addition to releasing secretin, acid exerts an important negative feedback control of gastrin release. Acidification of the antral mucosa below pH 3.5 inhibits gastrin release. Patients with atrophic gastritis, pernicious anemia, or other conditions characterized by the chronic decrease of acid-secreting cells and hyposecretion of acid may have extremely high serum concentrations of gastrin because of the absence of this inhibitory mechanism.

There are several instances in which hormones alter the release of GI peptides. Secretin and glucagon, for example, both inhibit gastrin release. CCK has been shown to stimulate glucagon release, and all four GI hormones increase insulin secretion. Elevated serum calcium stimulates both gastrin and CCK release. It is doubtful whether any of these mechanisms, except the release of insulin by GIP, play a role in normal GI physiology. Some, however, may become important when circulating levels of hormones or calcium are altered by disease.

■ ACTIONS AND INTERACTIONS

The effects of pure GI hormones have been tested on almost every secretory, motor, and absorptive function of the GI tract. Each peptide has some action on almost every target tested. Even though large doses of hormone are sometimes necessary to produce an effect, either stimulatory or inhibitory, the fact that receptors for each hormone are present on most target tissues is demonstrated. To indicate the myriad activities possessed by these peptides, many of their actions are summarized in Table 1-2.

The important physiologic actions of the GI hormones are depicted in Table 1-3. Numerous guidelines have been proposed for determining whether an action is physiologic. The action should occur in response to endogenous hormone released by normal stimuli, that is, those present during a meal. In other words, an exogenous dose of hormone should produce the effect in question without elevating serum hormone

TABLE 1-2

Actions of gastrointestinal hormones

	Hormones				
Action	Gastrin	CCK	Secretin	GIP	Motilin
Acid secretion	S	S	I	I	
Gastric emptying	I	I	I	I	
Pancreatic HCO_3^- secretion	S	S	S	O	
Pancreatic enzyme secretion	S	S	S	O	
Bile HCO_3^- secretion	S	S	S	O	
Gallbladder contraction	S	S	S		
Gastric motility	S	S	I	I	S
Intestinal motility	S	S	I		S
Insulin release	S	S	S	S	
Mucosal growth	S	S	I		
Pancreatic growth	S	S	S		

S, Stimulates; I, inhibits; O, no effect; Blank spaces, not yet tested.

Important actions of gastrointestinal hormones

	Hormones				
Action	Gastrin	CCK	Secretin	GIP	Motilin
Acid secretion	S		I	I	
Pancreatic HCO_3^- secretion		S	S		
Pancreatic enzyme secretion		S			
Bile HCO_3^- secretion			S		
Gallbladder contraction		S			
Gastric emptying		I			
Insulin release				S	
Mucosal growth	S				
Pancreatic growth		S	S		
Gastric motility					S
Intestinal motility					S

S, Stimulates; I, inhibits.

levels above those produced by a meal. An acceptable guideline for exogenous infusion is the dose that produces 50% of the maximal response (D_{50}) of the primary action of the hormone. The hormone should be administered as a continuous intravenous infusion rather than as a single bolus because the latter produces transient, unphysiologically high serum levels.

The primary action of gastrin is the stimulation of gastric acid secretion. On a molar basis it is 1500 times more potent than histamine. In humans the D_{50} is 1 ng/kg•min. There is considerable debate about the role of gastrin in regulating the tone of the lower esophageal sphincter, with the bulk of evidence indicating no normal role for gastrin in the regulation.

One of the most important and recently discovered actions of GI hormones is their trophic activity. Gastrin stimulates synthesis of RNA, protein, and DNA, as well as growth of the mucosa of the small intestine, colon, and oxyntic gland area of the stomach. If most endogenous gastrin is removed by antrectomy, these tissues atrophy. Exogenous gastrin prevents the atrophy. Patients with tumors that constantly secrete gastrin exhibit hyperplasia and hypertrophy of the acid-secreting portion of the stomach. Gastrin also stimulates the growth of the **enterochromaffin-like** (ECL) **cells** of the stomach. Continued hypersecretion of gastrin results in ECL-cell hyperplasia, which may develop into carcinoid tumors. The trophic effects of gastrin are restricted to GI tissues and are counteracted by secretin. The trophic action of gastrin is a direct effect that can be demonstrated in tissue culture.

The primary effect of secretin is the stimulation of pancreatic fluid and bicarbonate secretion; one of the primary actions of CCK is the stimulation of pancreatic enzyme secretion. In addition, CCK has a physiologically important interaction in potentiating the primary effect of secretin. Thus CCK greatly increases the pancreatic bicarbonate response to low circulating levels of secretin.

Both CCK and secretin also stimulate the growth of the exocrine pancreas. CCK exerts a stronger effect than does secretin, but the combination of the two hormones produces a potentiated response in rats that is truly remarkable. It is likely that the effects of these two hormones on pancreatic growth are as important as their effects on pancreatic secretion.

In addition to its effects on the pancreas, secretin stimulates biliary secretion of fluid and bicarbonate. This action also is shared by CCK, but secretin is the most potent choleretic of the GI hormones. In dogs, secretin is a potent inhibitor of gastrin-stimulated acid secretion. This action, however, probably is not physiologically important in humans. The ability of secretin to inhibit acid secretion may be important in some human diseases, however, and the student should be aware of this action. Secretin has been nicknamed "nature's antacid," for almost all its actions reduce the amount of acid in the duodenum. The only known exception to this general statement is its pepsigogic activity. Secretin is second only to ACh in promoting pepsinogen secretion from the chief cells of the stomach. Under normal circumstances only small amounts of secretin are released, making it doubtful whether secretin stimulates pepsin secretion physiologically.

In addition to its physiologic actions on pancreatic and biliary secretion, CCK regulates gallbladder contraction and gastric emptying. CCK is the most potent regulator of gallbladder contraction of the gastrointestinal peptides. It is approximately 100 times more effective than the gastrin tetrapeptide in contracting the gallbladder. CCK causes significant inhibition of gastric emptying in doses equal to the D_{50} of pancreatic secretion. Gastrin also inhibits gastric emptying, but the effective dose is about 6 times the D_{50} for stimulation of acid secretion by gastrin. This is the type of data that support conclusions that CCK physiologically inhibits gastric emptying and that gastrin does not.

There are several peptides, including secretin and GIP, that are enterogastrones. GIP was originally discovered because of its ability to inhibit gastric acid secretion and may well have been the original enterogastrone described by Ivy and Farrell in 1925. This action has not been established as physiologically significant in the innervated stomach. GIP, however, is a strong stimulator of insulin release and is responsible for the observation that an oral glucose load releases more insulin and is metabolized more rapidly than an equal amount of glucose administered intravenously.

Motilin stimulates the so-called migrating motility or myoelectric complex that moves through the stomach and small bowel every 90 minutes in the fasted gastrointestinal tract. Its cyclical release into the blood is inhibited by the ingestion of a meal. This is the only known function of this peptide.

■ CANDIDATE HORMONES

Earlier in this chapter certain peptides isolated from digestive tract tissue have been mentioned that may, at a later date, qualify as hormones. These often are referred to as candidate or putative hormones. Many have been proposed, but interest is greatest for those listed in Table 1-4. Enteroglucagon belongs to the secretin family. **Pancreatic polypeptide** and **peptide YY** (tyrosine-tyrosine) belong to the same family and are unrelated to either gastrin or secretin.

Pancreatic polypeptide was first identified as a minor impurity in insulin. It was then isolated and found to be a linear peptide with 36 amino acid residues. From a physiologic viewpoint the most important action of pancreatic polypeptide is the inhibition of both pancreatic bicarbonate and enzyme secretion, because this effect has the lowest dose requirement. Most constituents of a meal release pancreatic polypeptide, and the serum levels reached are sufficient to inhibit pancreatic secretion. Because the peak rate of pancreatic secretion during a meal is less than the maximal rate that can be achieved with exoge-

T A B L E   1 - 4

Candidate hormones

Peptide	Released by	Actions
Pancreatic polypeptide	Protein Fat Glucose	$\downarrow$ Pancreatic HCO_3^- and enzyme secretion
Peptide YY	Fat	$\downarrow$ Gastric secretion $\downarrow$ Gastric emptying
Enteroglucagon	Hexose Fat	$\downarrow$ Gastric secretion $\downarrow$ Gastric emptying $\uparrow$ Insulin release

$\downarrow$, Inhibits; $\uparrow$, stimulates.

nous stimuli, it is possible that pancreatic polypeptide modulates this response under normal conditions. Before it can be concluded that pancreatic polypeptide is responsible for the physiologic inhibition of pancreatic secretion, it must be shown that this actually occurs and that pancreatic polypeptide is the agent involved. The fact that the peptide is located in the pancreas and cannot be removed without also removing its target organ makes this evidence difficult to obtain.

Peptide YY was discovered in porcine small intestine and named for its amino- and carboxyl-terminal amino acid residues—both tyrosines. Of its 36 amino acid residues, 18 are identical to those of pancreatic polypeptide. Peptide YY is released by meals, and especially by fat. It may appear in plasma in concentrations sufficient to inhibit gastric secretion and emptying, and thus qualify as an enterogastrone. Its effects do not appear to be direct in that it does not inhibit secretion in response to gastrin or histamine. It does inhibit neurally stimulated secretion, but its final status as an enterogastrone has not been determined.

The enteroglucagons are products of the same gene processed in the pancreatic alpha cell to form glucagon. The intestinal L cell makes three forms of glucagon, one of which, **glucagon-like peptide-1** (GLP-1), may have important physiologic actions. This 30–amino acid peptide is a potent insulin releaser, even in the absence of hyperglycemia, and also inhibits gastric secretion and emptying. The significance of its effects remains to be established.

■ **NEUROCRINES**

Originally all GI peptides were believed to originate from endocrine cells and, therefore, to be either hormones or candidate hormones. With the advent of sophisticated immunocytochemical techniques for tissue localization of peptides, it became apparent that many were contained within the nerves of the gut.

Numerous peptides have been found in both the brain and the digestive tract mucosa. The first of these to be isolated was substance P, which in the GI tract has the property of stimulating intestinal motility and gallbladder contraction. The only other peptide isolated from both the brain and gut and known to have identical structures in both sites is neurotensin. Neurotensin increases blood glucose by stimulating glycogenolysis and glucagon release and inhibit-

T A B L E   1 - 5

Neurocrines

Peptide	Location	Actions
VIP	Mucosa and muscle of gut	Relaxation of gut smooth muscle
GRP or bombesin	Gastric mucosa	↑ Gastrin release
Enkephalins	Mucosa and muscle of gut	↑ Smooth muscle tone

↑, Stimulates.

ing insulin release. Other peptides have been isolated from one site and identified by radioimmunoassay in the other. These include motilin, CCK, and VIP, which were first isolated from the gut. Enkephalin, somatostatin, and thyrotropin-releasing factor were first isolated from the brain and later found in the gut. Gastrin, VIP, somatostatin, and enkephalin also are present in the nerves of the gut.

There are probably three peptides that function physiologically in the gut as neurocrines. These are listed in Table 1-5. Originally investigators thought VIP was found in gut endocrine cells. It is now known to be localized within the gut exclusively to nerves. It physiologically mediates the relaxation of GI smooth muscle. Smooth muscle is innervated by VIP-containing fibers, and VIP is released during relaxation. VIP relaxes smooth muscle, and VIP antiserum blocks neurally induced relaxation. In addition, there is strong evidence that VIP physiologically mediates relaxation of smooth muscle in blood vessels and thus may be responsible for vasodilation. Besides these effects, VIP has many of the actions of its relatives, secretin and GIP, when injected into the bloodstream. It stimulates pancreatic secretion, inhibits gastric secretion, and stimulates intestinal secretion.

Numerous biologically active peptides have been isolated from amphibian skin and later found to have mammalian counterparts. One of these, called bombesin, after the species of frog from which it was isolated, is a potent releaser of gastrin. The mammalian counterpart of bombesin is gastrin-releasing peptide (GRP) and has been found in the nerves of the gastric mucosa. GRP is released by vagal stimulation and mediates the vagal release of gastrin. Luminal protein digestion products also may stimulate gastrin release through a GRP-mediated mechanism.

Two pentapeptides isolated from pig and calf brains activate opiate receptors and are called enkephalins. They are identical except that the carboxy-terminal amino acid is methionine in one and leucine in the other. These compounds are present in nerves within both the smooth muscle and the mucosa of the gastrointestinal tract. Opiate receptors on circular smooth muscle cells mediate contraction; and leu-enkephalin and met-enkephalin cause contraction of the lower esophageal, pyloric, and ileocecal sphincters. The enkephalins function physiologically at these sites and also may be an intricate part of the peristaltic mechanism. The effect of opiates on intestinal motility is to slow transit of material through the gut. These peptides also inhibit intestinal secretion. The combination of these actions probably accounts for the effectiveness of opiates in treating diarrhea.

■ PARACRINES

Paracrines are like hormones in that they are released from endocrine cells. They are similar to neurocrines because they interact with receptors close to the point of their release. The biologic significance of an endocrine can be assessed by correlating physiologic events with changes in blood levels of the hormone in question. Because the area of release of both paracrines and neurocrines is restricted, there are no comparable methods for proving the biologic significance of one of these agents. Current experiments examine the effects of specific pharmacologic blockers or antisera directed toward these substances. In vitro perfused organs are also useful in examining paracrine mediators. These systems allow the investigator to collect and assay small volumes of venous perfusate for the agent in question.

One GI peptide, **somatostatin,** functions physiologically as a paracrine to inhibit gastrin release and gastric acid secretion. Somatostatin was first isolated from the hypothalamus as a growth hormone release inhibitory factor. It has since been shown to exist throughout the gastric and duodenal mucosa and the pancreas in high concentrations and to inhibit the release of all gut hormones. Somatostatin mediates the inhibition of gastrin release occurring when the antral mucosa is acidified. Somatostatin also directly inhibits acid secretion from the parietal cells. These are important physiologic actions of this peptide.

Histamine is a second important paracrine agent. Produced in ECL cells by the decarboxylation of histidine, histamine is released by gastrin and then stimulates acid secretion from the gastric parietal cells. Histamine also potentiates the action of gastrin and acetylcholine on acid secretion. This is why the histamine H_2-receptor blocking drugs like cimetidine (Tagamet) and ranitidine (Zantac) are effective inhibitors of acid secretion.

■ CLINICAL APPLICATIONS

Non–beta cell tumors of the pancreas or duodenal tumors may produce gastrin and continually release it into the blood. This disease is known as gastrinoma or Zollinger-Ellison syndrome. The tumors are small and difficult to define and resect; and if metastasizing, they grow slowly. Gastrin is released from these tumors at a high spontaneous rate that is not altered by feeding. The hypergastrinemia results in hypersecretion of gastric acid through two mechanisms. First, the trophic action of gastrin leads to increased parietal cell mass and acid secretory capacity. Second, increased serum gastrin levels constantly stimulate secretion from the hyperplastic mucosa. The complications of this disease—fulminant peptic ulceration, diarrhea, steatorrhea, and hypokalemia—are caused by the presence of large amounts of acid in the small bowel. The continual presence of acid in the duodenum overwhelms the neutralizing ability of the pancreas, erodes the mucosa, and produces ulcers. In large amounts gastrin inhibits absorption of fluid and electrolytes by the intestine, thereby adding to the large volumes of fluid (up to 10 L/day) entering the intestine. Increased intestinal transit probably also contributes to the diarrhea. Steatorrhea is produced by inactivation of pancreatic lipase and precipitation of bile salts at low luminal pH. Because the tumors are difficult to resect and the clinical manifestations are caused by hypersecretion of gastric acid, the preferred surgical treatment is removal of the target organ (the stomach). Although gastrin levels remain elevated, total gastrectomy stops the ulceration and diarrhea. This disease also may be treated nonsurgically with some of the powerful new drugs that inhibit acid secretion. (See Chapter 8.)

The only other clinical condition attributed to the overproduction of a GI peptide concerns VIP. Pancreatic cholera or watery diarrhea syndrome is a frequently lethal disease resulting from the secretion of a peptide by a pancreatic islet cell tumor. This peptide is a potent stimulus for intestinal secretion of the fluid and electrolytes that produce the copious diarrhea. VIP has been identified in both tumor tissue and the serum of these patients. Its ability to stimulate cholera-like fluid secretion from the intestine indicates that it is responsible for this disease.

■ CLINICAL TESTS

Gastrin is routinely measured by radioimmunoassay in clinical laboratories. Normal serum gastrin values must be set by each laboratory for its particular assay. If the normal mean serum gastrin concentration is taken as 50 pg/ml, serum gastrin in fasting patients with gastrinoma usually will exceed 200 pg/ml. The degree of overlap between patients with gastrinoma and those with ordinary duodenal ulcer disease means that specific tests are required to diagnose the gastrinoma.

The tests most widely used in the evaluation of hypergastrinemia include stimulation with protein meals, intravenous calcium infusion, and secretin infusion. Patients with Zollinger-Ellison syndrome may not release gastrin in detectable amounts in response to food. This may be due to the low pH of gastric contents caused by ongoing acid secretion stimulated by preexisting high serum gastrin levels. Acid in the antrum inhibits gastrin release, and any gastrin that might be released would be difficult to detect against the already high serum levels.

Gastrinoma patients may have an exaggerated acid secretory response to calcium infusions caused by the release of gastrin from tumor tissue. This test is run by infusing 5 mg of ionizable calcium per kilogram per hour as calcium gluconate for 3 hours while simultaneously measuring acid secretion and collecting blood samples at hourly intervals for gastrin determination. Peak gastrin responses usually are obtained 3 hours after calcium infusion is begun. In most patients with gastrinoma, serum gastrin concentrations will at least double so that the gastrin values will be over 500 pg/ml. Patients with ordinary ulcer disease may show moderate increases in serum gastrin with calcium infusion, but absolute gastrin values after stimulation seldom exceed 200 to 300 pg/ml.

The most specific and easiest test to administer for gastrinoma is secretin injection. Secretin inhibits antral gastrin release and yet stimulates tumor gastrin release in almost all patients with gastrinoma. Secretin (1 U/kg) is given as a rapid intravenous injection and will cause a peak increase in serum gastrin 5 to 10 minutes later. In a patient with definitely increased basal serum gastrin and acid hypersecretion, a doubling of serum gastrin at 5 to 10 minutes strongly indicates the presence of a gastrinoma.

■ SUMMARY

1. The functions of the GI tract are regulated by mediators acting as hormones (endocrines), paracrines, or neurocrines.
2. Two chemically related families of peptides are responsible for much of the regulation of GI function. These are the gastrin-CCK peptides and a second group containing secretin, VIP, GIP, and glucagon.
3. The GI hormones are located in endocrine cells scattered throughout the mucosa and are released by chemicals in food, neural activity, or physical distention.
4. The GI peptides have many pharmacologic actions, but only a few of these are physiologically significant.
5. Gastrin, CCK, secretin, GIP, and motilin are important GI hormones.
6. Somatostatin and histamine have important functions as paracrine agents.
7. VIP, bombesin (GRP), and the enkephalins are released from nerves and mediate many important functions of the digestive tract.

■ **KEY WORDS AND CONCEPTS**

- Endocrines or hormones
- Paracrines
- Neurocrines
- Acetylcholine
- Secretin
- Gastrin
- Cholecystokinin
- Enterogastrone
- Gastric inhibitory peptide
- Motilin
- Gastrin II
- Vasoactive intestinal peptide
- Glucagon
- Enteroglucagon
- Little gastrin or G 17
- Big gastrin or G 34
- Amine precursor uptake decarboxylation
- Enterochromaffin-like cells
- Pancreatic polypeptide
- Peptide YY
- Glucagon-like peptide-1
- Somatostatin
- Histamine

■ **BIBLIOGRAPHY**

Dockray GJ: Physiology of enteric neuropeptides. In Johnson LR, editor: *Physiology of the gastrointestinal tract,* ed 3, New York, 1994, Raven Press.

Johnson LR: Regulation of gastrointestinal mucosal growth. In Johnson LR, editor: *Physiology of the gastrointestinal tract,* ed 3, New York, 1994, Raven Press.

Makhlouf GM, editor: *Handbook of physiology,* section 6, *The gastrointestinal system,* vol 2, *Neural and endocrine biology,* Bethesda, Md, 1989, American Physiological Society.

Pearse AGE, Takor T: Embryology of the diffuse neuroendocrine system and its relationship to the common peptides, *Fed Proc* 38:2288-2294, 1979.

Solcia E, Capella C, Buffa R, Usellini L, Fiocca R, Sessa F: Endocrine cells of the digestive system. In Johnson LR, editor: *Physiology of the gastrointestinal tract,* ed 2, New York, 1987, Raven Press.

Walsh JH: Gastrointestinal hormones. In Johnson LR, editor: *Physiology of the gastrointestinal tract,* ed 3, New York, 1994, Raven Press.

Walsh JH, Grossman MI: Gastrin, *N Engl J Med* 292:1324-1332; 1337-1384, 1975.

Walsh JH, Grossman MI: The Zollinger-Ellison syndrome, *Gastroenterology* 65:140-165, 1973.

Regulation

Nerves and Smooth Muscle

Norman W. Weisbrodt

Secretory, motility, and absorptive functions of the gastrointestinal (GI) system must be integrated to accomplish digestion and absorption of meals and to maintain homeostasis between meals. This integration is mediated by regulatory systems that monitor events within the body (primarily the GI tract) and in the external environment. The information then is processed such that appropriate commands to increase and/or decrease activities of the various organs are given. In all known cases, these commands are mediated through the actions of specific chemicals on target cells of the digestive organs. The manner in which these chemicals reach the target cells defines the various regulatory systems. In Chapter 1, the endocrine, paracrine, and neurocrine systems are discussed. In this chapter, the role of the nervous (neurocrine) system is considered in more detail.

Although the regulatory systems act to integrate activities of the GI system, most secretory, absorptive, and muscle cells possess intrinsic activities that give them a degree of autonomy. Thus, function arises out of the interaction of regulatory systems and local intrinsic properties. The basic intrinsic properties of each type of secretory and absorptive cell are discussed in sep-

arate chapters that deal with the secretion and absorption of specific chemicals. The basic properties and intrinsic activities of the smooth muscle cells are discussed in this chapter.

■ ANATOMY OF THE AUTONOMIC NERVOUS SYSTEM

The GI tract is innervated by the **autonomic nervous system** (ANS). It is called the ANS since we normally are not conscious of its activities nor do we exert any willful control over them. The ANS can be divided into the extrinsic nervous system and the intrinsic or enteric nervous system.

The **extrinsic nervous system** is in turn divided into the parasympathetic and the sympathetic branches (Figure 2-1). **Parasympathetic innervation** is supplied primarily by the vagus and pelvic nerves. Long preganglionic axons arise from cell bodies within the medulla of the brain and the sacral region of the spinal cord. These preganglionic nerves enter the various organs of the gastrointestinal tract where they synapse mainly with cells of the enteric nervous system. In addition, these same nerve bundles contain many afferent nerves whose receptors lie within the various tissues of the gut. These

15

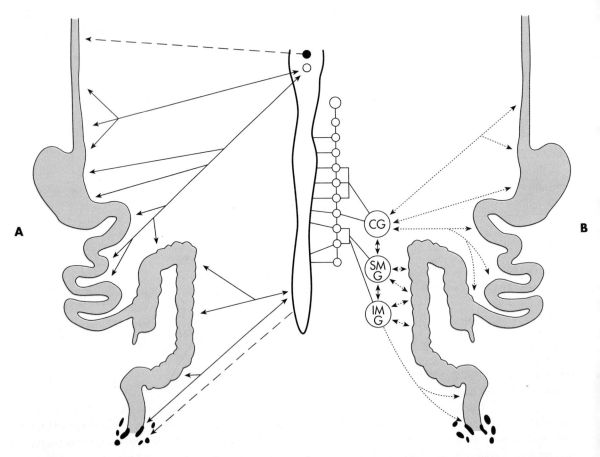

Figure 2-1 ■ Extrinsic branches of the ANS. A, Parasympathetic. Dashed lines indicate the cholinergic innervation of striated muscle in the esophagus and external anal sphincter. Solid lines indicate the afferent and preganglionic efferent innervation of the rest of the GI tract. B, Sympathetic. Solid lines denote the afferent and preganglionic efferent connections between the spinal cord and the prevertebral ganglia (*CG,* celiac; *SMG,* superior mesenteric; *IMG,* inferior mesenteric). Dashed lines indicate the afferent and postganglionic efferent innervation.

nerves project to the brain and spinal cord to provide sensory input for integration.

Sympathetic innervation is supplied by nerves that run between the spinal cord and the prevertebral ganglia and between these ganglia and the organs of the gut. Preganglionic efferent fibers arise within the cord and end in the prevertebral ganglia. Postganglionic fibers from these ganglia then innervate primarily elements

of the enteric nervous system. Few fibers end directly on secretory, absorptive, or muscle cells. Afferent fibers also are present within the sympathetic division. These nerves project back to the prevertebral ganglia and/or the spinal cord. Thus an abundance of sensory information is available.

Elements of the **intrinsic or enteric nervous system** are grouped into several anatomi-

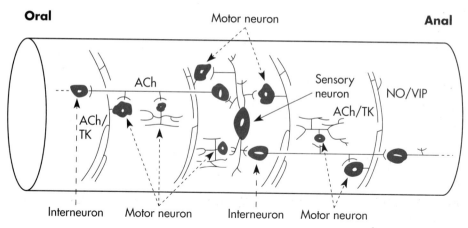

Oral — Motor neuron — **Anal**

ACh — Sensory neuron — NO/VIP — ACh/TK

ACh/TK

Interneuron — Motor neuron — Interneuron — Motor neuron

Figure 2-2 ■ Schematic of a horizontal section through the wall of the intestine at the level of the myenteric plexus, showing examples of neuronal circuits intrinsic to the intestine. Sensory neurons provide synaptic inputs to motor neurons and to interneurons. Interneurons connect with other interneurons in chains and also innervate motor neurons. Most regions of the GI tract contain multiple overlapping circuits of this type, with extensive convergence and divergence of connections. Some of the transmitters that have been localized to intrinsic nerves are indicated (*ACh*, acetylcholine; *TK*, tachykinins; *VIP*, vasoactive intestinal peptide; *NO*, nitric oxide). Many pathways are yet to be mapped. Not shown are the extrinsic nerves that provide synaptic input to the intrinsic nerves and that provide sensory information to neurons in extrinsic ganglia, the spinal cord, and the brain. (Adapted from Furness JB, Bornstein JC, Pompolo S, Young HM, Kunze WAA, Kelly H: The circuitry of the enteric nervous system, *Neurogastroenterol Mot* 6:241-253, 1994.)

cally distinct networks, of which the **myenteric and submucosal plexuses** are the most prominent. These plexuses consist of nerve cell bodies, axons, dendrites, and nerve endings. Processes from the neurons of the plexuses do not just innervate target cells such as smooth muscle, secretory cells, and absorptive cells. They also connect to sensory receptors and interdigitate with processes from other neurons located both inside and outside the plexus. Thus pathways within the enteric nervous system can be multisynaptic, and integration of activities can take place entirely within the enteric nervous system (Figure 2-2).

There are a large number of chemicals that serve as **neurocrines** within the ANS. Several of these chemicals have been localized within specific pathways, and a few have defined physiologic roles. Most of the extrinsic, preganglionic,

efferent fibers contain **acetylcholine** (ACh). This transmitter exerts its action on neurons contained within the prevertebral ganglia and the enteric nervous system. **Norepinephrine** is found in many nerve endings of the postganglionic efferent nerves of the sympathetic nervous system. This transmitter also exerts its effects primarily on neurons of the enteric nervous system. Within the enteric nervous system, ACh, **serotonin, vasoactive intestinal peptide** (VIP), **nitric oxide,** and **somatostatin** have been localized to interneurons; ACh and the tachykinins (such as **substance P**) have been localized to nerves that are excitatory to the muscle; and VIP and nitric oxide have been localized to inhibitory nerves to the muscle. In many instances, more than one transmitter can be localized to the same nerve. Mapping neural circuits within the extrinsic and enteric nervous system and elucidating their functions is far from complete.

■ NEUROHUMORAL REGULATION OF GASTROINTESTINAL FUNCTION

Although it is convenient to discuss the ANS and the endocrine/paracrine systems separately, it is important to understand that they do not function independently of one another. Rather, the regulatory systems interact to control secretion, absorption, and motility. Specific examples of such regulation are given in the following chap-

ters. (See Figures 8-10 and 9-7 for examples.) A general scheme of the interaction is depicted in Figure 2-3. The target cells, be they secretory, absorptive, or smooth muscle cells, have a certain resting output that is modulated by both neurally released and humorally delivered chemicals. These chemicals are released from nerve endings and glandular cells in response to various stimuli that act upon specific receptors. The sources of these stimuli can be either in the environment or within the body. For example, sighting and smelling appetizing food alters many aspects of

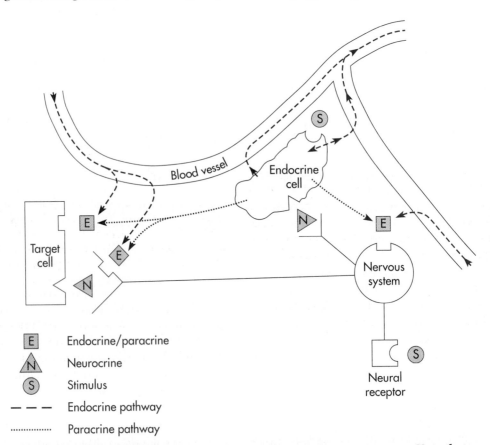

E	Endocrine/paracrine
N	Neurocrine
S	Stimulus
- - -	Endocrine pathway
....	Paracrine pathway

Figure 2-3 ■ Pathways by which integration of the regulatory systems can occur. Note that most target cells or tissues possess intrinsic activities that are modulated by specific chemicals acting on specific receptors. These chemicals come from nerve endings and endocrine cells. Note also that these same chemicals, as well as the products of the target cells, can alter activities of the nerves and endocrine cells themselves.

GI function, as does the presence of many food-stuffs and products of digestion within the lumen of the stomach and intestine. In many cases, the stimuli result from the secretory and motor functions of the target cells themselves. Whatever their source, these stimuli initiate inputs that are integrated in the neural and endocrine systems in such a way that the output of target cells is modulated appropriately. Thus there are examples of neural activity causing the release of hormones, of hormones modulating neural activity, and of effector cell activity being influenced simultaneously by neural and hormonal activities.

■ ANATOMY OF THE SMOOTH MUSCLE CELL

The contractile tissue of the GI tract is made up of **smooth muscle cells,** except in the pharynx, the orad third of the esophagus, and the external anal sphincter. The smooth muscle cells found in each region of the GI tract exhibit functional and structural differences. These special features are considered in the following chapters. However, certain basic properties are common to all smooth muscle cells. The cells are small compared with skeletal muscle, being some 4 to 10 μm wide and 50 to 200 μm long. A distinguishing feature of these cells is that the contractile elements are not arranged in orderly sarcomeres as in skeletal muscle (Figure 2-4). Thus the cells have no striations. The contractile proteins, actin and myosin, are present in myofilaments. Actin, along with tropomyosin, constitutes the thin filaments, whereas myosin constitutes the thick filaments. Compared with skeletal muscle, smooth muscle contains less myosin, much more actin, and little if any troponin. The apparent ratio of thin to thick filaments in smooth muscles is 12 to 18:1, rather than 2:1 as in skeletal muscle. In addition to the thick and thin filaments, smooth muscle cells contain a third network of filaments that form an internal "skeleton." These intermediate filaments, along

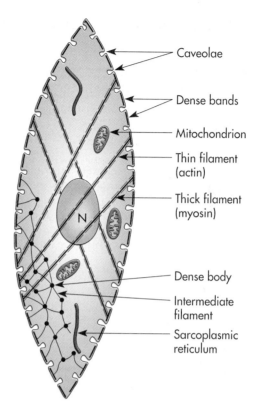

Figure 2-4 ■ Intracellular structural specializations of a smooth muscle cell. (Adapted from Schiller LR: Motor function of the stomach. In Sleisenger MH, Fordtran JS, editors: *Gastrointestinal disease,* Philadelphia, 1983, WB Saunders, pp 521-540.)

with their associated dense bodies, may serve as anchor points for the contractile filaments.

Smooth muscle cells of the GI tract are grouped into branching bundles or **fasciae** that are surrounded by connective tissue sheets. These fasciae, organized into muscular coats, can serve as the effector units because smooth muscle cells of the gut are mostly of the "unitary" type (Figure 2-5). Individual cells are functionally coupled to one another so that contractions of a bundle of muscle are synchronous. In most tissues, this coupling is due to actual fusion of apposing membranes in the form of gap junctions

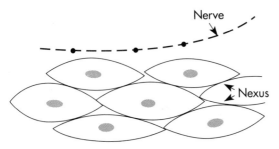

Figure 2-5 ■ **Anatomic features of "unitary" smooth muscle. Neurotransmitter is released from varicosities along the nerve trunk. Other chemicals arrive via endocrine and paracrine routes. The influence of these substances on one muscle cell is then transmitted to other cells via nexuses.**

or nexuses. These junctions serve as areas of low resistance for the spread of excitation from one cell to another. Not every smooth muscle cell is innervated. Nerve axons enter the muscle bundles and release neurotransmitters from swellings along their length. These swellings are usually some distance from the muscle cells so that no discrete neuromuscular junctions exist. Thus the neurotransmitters probably act on only a few of the cells. The influence of the transmitters then must be communicated from one smooth muscle cell to the next.

■ SMOOTH MUSCLE CONTRACTION

There is a remarkable heterogeneity in the time-course of contractions among smooth muscles in the gastrointestinal tract. Some muscles, such as those found in the body of the esophagus, the small bowel, and the gastric antrum, contract and relax in a matter of seconds (**phasic contractions**). Other smooth muscles, such as those found in the lower esophageal sphincter, the orad stomach, and the ileocecal and internal anal sphincters, show sustained contractions that last from minutes to hours. These muscles exhibit what are called **tonic contractions.** As discussed in the following chapters, the type of

contraction, whether phasic or tonic, is governed by the smooth muscle cells themselves. It does not depend upon neural or hormonal input. Neurocrines, endocrines, and paracrines are important because they modulate the basic contractile activity, so that the amplitude of the contractions of phasic muscles varies and the tone of the tonic muscles increases or decreases.

As in striated muscle, contractile activity of smooth muscle, especially those that contract phasically, is modulated by fluctuating levels of free intracellular **calcium.** At low levels ($<10^{-7}$ M) of calcium, interaction of the contractile proteins does not occur. At higher levels of calcium, proteins interact and contractions occur. The prevailing theory to explain how calcium brings about contraction is that the calcium, combined with the calcium-binding protein calmodulin, activates a protein kinase that brings about the specific phosphorylation of one of the components of myosin (Figure 2-6). Myosin in its phosphorylated form then interacts with actin to cause contraction, which is fueled by the splitting of **adenosine triphosphate** (ATP). When the intracellular levels of calcium fall, the myosin is dephosphorylated by a specific phosphatase. This brings about a cessation of the interaction between the contractile proteins and muscle relaxation. In smooth muscles that contract tonically, the exact mechanism for the maintenance of tone is not known. What is known is that tone can be maintained at low levels of phosphorylation of myosin and at low levels of ATP utilization.

The exact source of the calcium that participates in the contractile process is not certain and appears to vary from one muscle to another. In many muscles (e.g., muscle from the body of the esophagus) calcium enters the cells from the extracellular fluid or from pools of calcium that are tightly bound to the smooth muscle cell membranes or contained in caveolae (Figure 2-4). Influx of calcium from these sites is regulated by permeability changes of the membrane that also

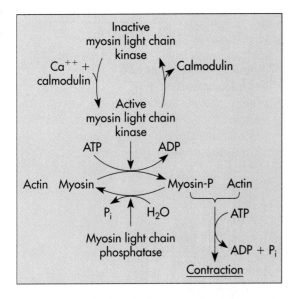

Figure 2-6 ■ Biochemical events in smooth muscle contraction. An increase in the levels of Ca⁺⁺ activates an enzyme (myosin light chain kinase), which phosphorylates myosin. Phosphorylated myosin *(myosin-P)* interacts with actin to cause muscle contraction. When Ca⁺⁺ levels fall, the kinase becomes inactive and the activity of myosin light chain phosphatase dominates. Myosin-P is dephosphorylated and the muscle relaxes.

cause characteristic electrical activities (see below). In other muscles (e.g., muscle from the lower esophageal sphincter) calcium is sequestered in intracellular structures called the sarcoplasmic reticulum (Figure 2-4) and is released in response to electrical events of the plasma membrane and/or to agonist-induced increases in inositol trisphosphate. In addition to these sources for calcium, mechanisms also exist for the expulsion of calcium from the cells and for reuptake into the sarcoplasmic reticulum.

Increases in free intracellular calcium most often are related to electrical activities of the smooth muscle cell membranes. In phasically active muscle, calcium enters the cell by way of voltage-dependent calcium channels. When these are activated, rapid transients in membrane po-

tential called **action or spike potentials** occur (Figure 5-6). In many phasic muscles these spike potentials do not arise from a stable resting membrane potential. Rather, they are superimposed on relatively slow (3 to 12 cycles/min) but regular oscillations in membrane potential. These potential changes, called **slow waves,** do not in themselves cause significant contractions. However, they set the timing for when spike potentials can occur, since spikes are seen only during the peak of depolarization of the slow wave. The genesis of slow waves has not been elucidated, despite intense investigation. The most recent hypothesis is that the oscillations originate in specialized cells called **interstitial cells of Cajal.** These distinct cells are heavily innervated and form gap junctions with smooth muscle cells.

Both slow waves and spike potentials are inherent to the smooth muscle cells themselves. Slow waves are extremely regular and are only minimally influenced by neural or hormonal activities. They are influenced by body temperature and metabolic activity. The higher the activity, the higher the frequency of slow waves. On the other hand, the occurrence of spike potentials depends heavily upon neural and hormonal activities.

An excitatory endocrine, paracrine, or neurocrine will act on a receptor on the smooth muscle cell membrane to induce spike potentials in those cells and in adjacent cells that are coupled to one another. The spike potentials lead to an increase in intercellular free Ca⁺⁺ levels. The Ca⁺⁺ then acts via myosin light chain kinase to induce **contraction.** On the other hand, an inhibitory mediator will act with its receptor on that same membrane. In this case, however, the response will be an inhibition of spike potentials and/or a hyperpolarization of the cell membrane. This results in a decrease in intracellular free Ca⁺⁺ and subsequent **relaxation.** The interplay of these excitatory and inhibitory mediators on the basal activity of the muscle determines the motility functions of the various organs of the gut.

■ SUMMARY

1. The regulation of GI function results from an interplay of neural and hormonal influences on effector cells that have intrinsic activities.

2. The GI tract is innervated by the ANS, which is composed of nerves that are extrinsic and nerves that are intrinsic to the tract.

3. Extrinsic nerves are distributed to the GI tract through both parasympathetic and sympathetic pathways.

4. Intrinsic nerves are grouped into several nerve plexuses, with the myenteric and submucosa plexuses being the most prominent. Nerves in the plexuses receive input from receptors within the GI tract and from extrinsic nerves. This input can be integrated within the intrinsic nerves such that coordinated activities can be effected.

5. Acetylcholine is one of the major excitatory neurotransmitters, and nitric oxide and VIP are two of the major inhibitory neurotransmitters at effector cells. Serotonin and somatostatin are two important neurotransmitters of intrinsic interneurons.

6. Striated muscle comprises the musculature of the pharynx, the orad half of the esophagus, and the external anal sphincter. Smooth muscle comprises the musculature of the rest of the GI tract.

7. Adjacent smooth muscle cells are electrically coupled to one another and contract synchronously when stimulated. Some smooth muscles contract tonically, whereas others contract phasically.

8. In phasically active muscle, stimulation induces a rise in intracellular calcium, which in turn induces phosphorylation of the 20,000-dalton light chain of myosin. ATP is split and the muscle contracts as the phosphorylated myosin interacts with actin. Calcium levels fall, myosin is dephosphorylated, and relaxation occurs. In tonically active muscles, contraction can be maintained at low levels of phosphorylation and ATP utilization.

■ KEY WORDS AND CONCEPTS

- Autonomic nervous system
- Extrinsic nervous system
- Parasympathetic innervation
- Sympathetic innervation
- Intrinsic or enteric nervous system
- Myenteric and submucosal plexuses
- Neurocrines
- Acetylcholine
- Norepinephrine
- Serotonin
- Vasoactive intestinal peptide
- Nitric oxide
- Somatostatin
- Substance P
- Smooth muscle cells
- Fasciae
- Phasic contractions
- Tonic contractions
- Calcium
- Adenosine triphosphate
- Action or spike potentials
- Slow waves
- Interstitial cells of Cajal
- Contraction
- Relaxation

■ BIBLIOGRAPHY

Furness JB, Bornstein JC: The enteric nervous system and its extrinsic connections. In Yamada T, editor: *Textbook of gastroenterology*, vol 1, ed 2, Philadelphia, 1995, JB Lippincott.

Gabella G: Structure of muscles and nerves in the gastrointestinal tract. In Johnson LR, editor: *Physiology of the gastrointestinal tract*, vol 1, ed 3, New York, 1994, Raven Press.

Murphy RA: Smooth muscle. In Berne RM, Levy MN, editors: *Physiology*, ed 3, St Louis, 1993, Mosby–Year Book.

Roman C, Gonella J: Extrinsic control of digestive tract motility. In Johnson LR, editor: *Physiology of the gastrointestinal tract*, vol 1, ed 2, New York, 1987, Raven Press.

Wood JD: Physiology of the enteric nervous system. In Johnson LR, editor: *Physiology of the gastrointestinal tract*, vol 1, ed 3, New York, 1994, Raven Press.

Swallowing

Norman W. Weisbrodt

The movement of food through the gastrointestinal (GI) tract beings with its **oral ingestion.** Once food has been savored, mixed with saliva, and reduced in particle size through the process of chewing, it is propelled to the stomach through the process of swallowing. Swallowing is almost purely a motility function. Little digestion and absorption takes place, in part because the transport of material into the stomach takes only seconds.

The process of swallowing involves the integrated contractile activities of the oral cavity, pharynx, esophagus, and orad portion of the stomach. It is initiated by propulsion of material into the oropharynx primarily by movements of the **tongue.** The portion to be swallowed is separated from other material in the mouth so it lies in a chamber created by placing the tip of the tongue against the hard palate (Figure 3-1, *A*). It is propelled by elevation and retraction of the tongue against the palate. As the material passes from the **oral cavity** into the **oropharynx,** the **nasopharynx** is closed by movement of the soft palate and contraction of the superior constrictor muscles of the pharynx (Figure 3-1, *B*). Simultaneously, respiration is inhibited and contraction of the laryngeal muscles closes the

glottis and raises the **larynx.** The bolus is propelled through the pharynx by a **peristaltic contraction** that begins in the superior constrictor and progresses through the middle and inferior constrictor muscles of the **pharynx** (Figure 3-1, *C*). These contractions, along with relaxation of the **upper esophageal sphincter** (UES) propel the bolus into the esophagus (Figure 3-1, *D*).

The oral and pharyngeal phases of swallowing are rapid, taking less than 1 second. Swallowing can be initiated voluntarily. Once initiated, however, it proceeds as a coordinated involuntary reflex. Coordination is central in origin, and an area within the reticular formation of the brain stem has been identified as the **swallowing center.** Afferent impulses from the pharynx are directed toward this center, which serves to coordinate activity of other areas of the brain such as the nuclei of the trigeminal, facial, and hypoglossal nerves, as well as the nucleus ambiguus (Figure 3-2). Efferent impulses from the center are distributed to the pharynx via nerves from the nucleus ambiguus. The impulses appear to be sequential, so the pharyngeal musculature is activated in a proximal-to-distal manner. This sequencing accounts for the peristaltic nature of

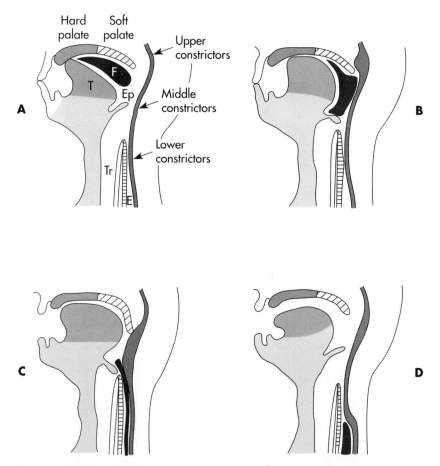

Figure 3-1 ■ Oral and pharyngeal events during swallowing. **A,** The bolus *(F)* to be swallowed is propelled into the pharynx by placement of the tongue *(T)* on the roof of the hard palate. **B,** Further propulsion is caused by movement of the more distal regions of the tongue against the palate. Contraction of the upper constrictors of the pharynx and movement of the soft palate separate the oropharynx from the nasopharynx. **C,** Propulsion through the UES is accomplished by contraction of the middle and lower constrictors of the pharynx and by relaxation of the cricopharyngeal muscle. Upward movement of the glottis and downward movement of the epiglottis *(Ep)* seal off the trachea *(Tr).* **D,** The bolus is now in the esophagus *(E)* and is propelled into the stomach by a peristaltic contraction.

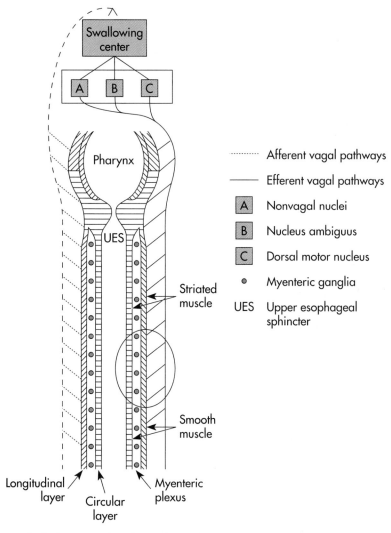

Figure 3-2 ■ **Control of pharyngeal and esophageal peristalsis. Sensory input from the pharynx activates an area in the medulla (the *swallowing center*). This center serves to coordinate activation of the vagal nuclei with other centers such as the respiratory centers. Muscles of the pharynx and striated areas of the esophagus are activated by the center via the nucleus ambiguus. Areas of the smooth muscle are activated via the dorsal motor nucleus. Peristalsis is due to sequential activation of the muscles of the pharynx and esophagus by sequential neural impulses from the center. The area enclosed within the circle is shown in more detail in Figure 3-4.**

the pharyngeal contractions. The center also appears to interact with other areas of the brain involved with respiration and speech. Ablation of the swallowing center produces loss of the pharyngeal component of swallowing.

■ ESOPHAGEAL PERISTALSIS

The **esophagus** propels material from the pharynx to the stomach. This propulsion is accomplished by coordinated contractions of the muscular layers of the body of the esophagus. Because a large segment of the esophagus is located in the thorax, where the pressure is lower than in the pharynx and stomach, the esophagus also must withstand entry of air and gastric contents. The barrier functions of the esophagus are accomplished by the presence of sphincters at each end of the organ.

Anatomically the esophageal muscle is arranged in two layers: an inner layer with the muscle fibers organized in a circular axis and an outer layer with the fibers organized in a longitudinal axis. The UES consists of a thickening of the circular muscle and can be identified anatomically as the cricopharyngeal muscle. This muscle, like the musculature of the proximal third of the esophageal body, is striated. The distal third of the esophagus is composed of smooth muscle; although the terminal 1 to 2 cm of the musculature acts as a sphincter, no separate sphincter muscle can be identified anatomically. The middle third of the body of the esophagus is composed of a mixture of muscle types with a descending transition from striated to smooth fibers.

The events that occur in the esophagus between and during swallowing often are monitored by placing pressure-sensing devices at various levels in the esophageal lumen. Such devices indicate that between swallows both the UES and the **lower esophageal sphincter** (LES) are closed and the body of the esophagus is flaccid (Figure 3-3, *A*). At the upper end of the esophagus, a zone of 1 to 2 cm is detected where the pressure exceeds that on either side of the zone

by as much as 60 mm Hg. A zone of elevated pressure is also found at the lower end of the esophagus. The length of this zone may vary from several millimeters to a few centimeters, and the pressure may be 20 to 40 mm Hg higher than on either side. Pressures in the body of the esophagus are similar to those within the body cavity in which the esophagus lies. In the thorax the pressure varies with respiration, dropping with inspiration and rising with expiration. These fluctuations in pressure with respiration reverse below the diaphragm, and intraluminal esophageal pressure reflects intraabdominal pressure.

During a swallow the sphincters and the body of the esophagus act in a coordinated manner (Figure 3-3, *B*). Shortly before the distal pharyngeal muscles contract, the UES opens. Once the bolus passes, the sphincter closes and assumes its resting tone. The body of the esophagus undergoes a peristaltic contraction. This contraction begins just below the UES and occurs sequentially at progressively more distal segments to give the appearance of a contractile wave moving toward the stomach. After the contractile sequence passes, the esophageal muscle becomes flaccid again. Shortly before the peristaltic contraction reaches the LES, the sphincter relaxes. After passage of the bolus the sphincter contracts back to its resting level. Compared with the rapid events in the pharynx, esophageal peristalsis is slow. The peristaltic contraction moves down the esophagus at velocities ranging from 2 to 6 cm/s, and may take 10 seconds to reach the lower end of the esophagus.

When esophageal peristalsis is preceded by a pharyngeal phase, it is called **primary peristalsis.** Esophageal contractions, however, can occur in the absence of both oral and pharyngeal phases. This is called **secondary peristalsis** and is elicited when the esophagus is distended. Secondary peristalsis occurs if the primary contraction fails to empty the esophagus or when gastric contents reflux into the esophagus. Initiation of secondary peristaltic contractions is

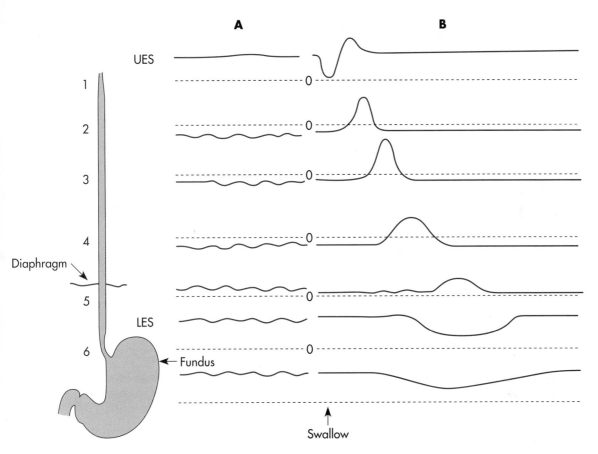

Figure 3-3 ■ Manometric recordings from the esophagus and orad stomach. Intraluminal pressures from the upper esophageal sphincter (*UES*), four areas of the esophagus, the lower esophageal sphincter (*LES*), and the gastric fundus are shown. A, Between swallows both the upper and the lower sphincters are closed, as indicated by the greater than atmospheric pressures recorded there. Pressures in the body of the esophagus reflect intrathoracic or intraabdominal pressures. Pressures in the fundus reflect intraabdominal pressure plus tonic contractions of the fundus. B, On swallowing, the upper sphincter relaxes before passage of the bolus. After bolus passage it contracts, to be followed by a peristaltic contraction in the body of the esophagus. To allow passage of the bolus into the stomach, the lower sphincter and the orad stomach relax before the peristaltic contraction reaches them.

involuntary and normally is not sensed.

The effect of esophageal peristalsis on bolus transport depends upon the physical properties of the bolus. If a person in an upright position swallows a liquid bolus, it actually reaches the stomach several seconds before the peristaltic contraction. Thus, although both sphincters must relax to allow transport of all materials, esophageal peristalsis is not always necessary. For most swallowed material, peristaltic contractions are essential for progression to the stomach, and repetitive secondary contractions often are required to sweep the bolus completely into the stomach.

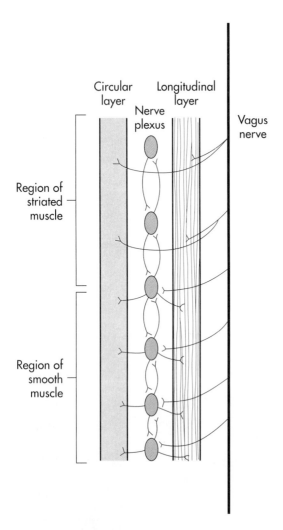

Figure 3-4 ■ Efferent innervation of the body of the esophagus. Special visceral somatic fibers directly innervate the striated muscle fibers of the circular and longitudinal muscle layers. Preganglionic fibers from the vagus innervate the ganglion cells of the intrinsic plexus. Fibers from the ganglion cells then innervate the smooth muscle cells of both layers. In addition, the ganglion cells have neural connections with one another.

Control of esophageal peristalsis is complex and not understood fully. Closure of the UES is maintained by the normal elasticity of the sphincteric structures as well as the active contraction of the cricopharyngeal muscle. Relaxation of the UES is coordinated with contraction of the pharyngeal musculature. As the larynx rises during the pharyngeal component of swallowing, the cricopharyngeal area is displaced. This displacement, along with relaxation of the cricopharyngeal muscle, allows the sphincter to open. Relaxation of the cricopharyngeal muscle is brought about by a suppression of nerve impulses from the swallowing center via activity of the nucleus ambiguus.

Contractions of the body of the esophagus are coordinated by both central and peripheral mechanisms. This region of the esophagus is innervated primarily by the vagus nerves. These nerves are partly of the somatic motor type, arising from the nucleus ambiguus, and partly of the visceral motor type, arising from the dorsal motor nucleus. The somatic motor nerves synapse directly with striated muscle fibers of the esophagus (Figure 3-4). The visceral motor nerves do not synapse directly with the smooth muscle cells but rather with nerve cell bodies that lie between the longitudinal and circular muscle layers. These local nerves, in turn, innervate the smooth muscle cells as well as communicate with one another along the length of the esophagus.

Central control originates within the swallowing center, which sends a series of sequential impulses to progressively more distal segments of the esophagus. This sequential activation results in a peristaltic contraction. The central nervous system does not totally control peristalsis, however. In smooth muscle areas of the esophagus, peristalsis can occur after bilateral cervical **vagotomy** (cutting of the vagus nerve). Furthermore, peristalsis can be induced in excised esophagi that have been placed in an organ bath. In these instances, peristalsis must be coordinated by the intrinsic nerve plexuses or the smooth muscle cells themselves.

The presence of secondary peristalsis indicates the importance of afferent input to the central and peripheral mechanisms controlling swallowing. Afferent input provided by distention of the esophagus not only initiates secondary peristalsis, it also affects the intensity of contractions. Variation in the size of the bolus being swallowed leads to a variation in the amplitude of esophageal contraction. Indeed, afferent stimulation appears so important that a peristaltic sequence may not occur unless a bolus is swallowed and elicits afferent stimulation. On the other hand, intense afferent stimulation, such as that provided by inflation of a balloon in the body of the esophagus, can inhibit the progression of peristaltic contractions past the balloon.

Contraction of the LES is regulated by the intrinsic properties of the smooth muscle fibers, as well as by neural and humoral influences. Smooth muscle from this area of the esophagus responds to passive stretching by contracting to oppose the stretch. This response does not depend on nervous activity. Thus the basic tone of the LES may be totally myogenic. Nevertheless, this tone is under a number of neural and humoral influences. For example, resting tone is increased by cholinergic agonists and by the GI hormone gastrin. Sphincteric tone is decreased by agents such as isoproterenol and prostaglandin E_1.

Transient relaxation of the LES during swallowing is mediated through enteric nerves. The enteric inhibitory nerves can be activated by stimulation of the vagus nerve and by distention of the body of the esophagus, thus activating orad enteric nerves. The neurochemical basis for this response is not known, although roles for both vasoactive intestinal peptide (VIP) and nitric oxide have been proposed.

■ RECEPTIVE RELAXATION OF THE STOMACH

Swallowing also involves the stomach. In terms of motility functions, the stomach can be divided into two major areas: the **orad portion,** which consists of the fundus and a portion of the body, and the **caudad portion,** which consists of the distal body and the antrum (Figure 3-5). These two regions have markedly different patterns of motility that are responsible, in part, for two major functions: accommodation of ingested material during swallowing, and regulation of gastric emptying. Accommodation is primarily attributable to activities of the orad region, whereas both regions are involved in the regulation of gastric emptying. (See Chapter 4.)

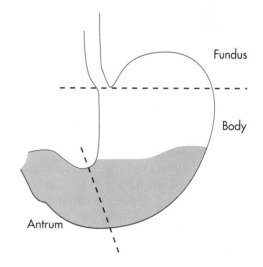

Figure 3-5 ■ Divisions of the stomach. For discussions of secretion the stomach is usually divided into fundus, body, and antrum. For discussions of motility it can be divided into an orad area and a caudad area. Stippling denotes the approximate extent of the caudad area.

During a swallow, the orad region of the stomach relaxes at about the same time as does the LES. Intraluminal pressures in both regions fall before arrival of the swallowed bolus because of active relaxation of the smooth muscle in both regions (Figure 3-3, *B*). After passage of the bolus, the pressure in the stomach returns to approximately what it was before the swallow. This process has been termed **receptive relaxation.** Because relaxation happens with each swallow, large volumes can be accommodated with a minimal rise in intragastric pressure. For example, the human stomach can accept 1600 ml of air with a rise in pressure of no more than 10 mm Hg.

Receptive relaxation is mediated by a nervous reflex that has its afferent and efferent pathways in the vagus nerve. If this nerve is transected, receptive relaxation is impaired and the stomach becomes less distensible. The neurotransmitters that mediate receptive relaxation are unknown, but again nitric oxide may be involved.

■ CLINICAL APPLICATIONS

Contractions of pharyngeal muscle are controlled solely by extrinsic nerves. Therefore certain neurologic diseases (such as cerebrovascular accident) can have an adverse effect on this phase of swallowing. Aspiration often occurs because contractions in the pharynx and UES are no longer coordinated. A similar clinical picture can be seen in diseases that affect striated muscle or the myoneural junction.

Diseases affecting the smooth muscle portion of the esophagus predictably cause abnormalities in peristalsis and in tone of the LES. In one disease, **achalasia,** the LES often fails to relax completely with swallowing. This may be coupled with loss of peristalsis in the esophageal body, complete absence of contractions, or appearance of simultaneous rather than sequential contractions, resulting in impaired transit. Patients with this disease have considerable difficulty swallowing, often aspirate retained esoph-

ageal content, and may become severely malnourished. This disorder has been attributed to abnormalities in the enteric nerves. In another disease, **diffuse esophageal spasm,** simultaneous contraction of long duration and high amplitude can occur. Affected individuals have difficulty swallowing and may complain of chest pain. Although not always symptomatic, abnormalities in the esophageal component of swallowing can occur as part of a variety of systemic diseases. Examples are diabetes mellitus, chronic alcoholism, and scleroderma.

Motor dysfunction can also play an important supporting role in the pathogenesis of other esophageal diseases. One common example is **acid injury to the esophageal mucosa,** which results from reflux of gastric contents. Often underlying this problem are abnormally low resting pressure and inappropriate transient relaxations of the LES, and poor or ineffective secondary peristalsis in the esophageal body. The causes of these motor abnormalities are unknown.

■ CLINICAL TESTS

Swallowing is assessed clinically by x-ray examination with barium and by esophageal manometry. In the x-ray study the patient swallows a bolus of liquid barium sulfate. This material is radiopaque and thus can be observed fluoroscopically and recorded on the x-ray film as it traverses the esophagus, thereby providing a qualitative description of motor events in both the pharynx and the esophagus.

If a more detailed description of events is required or there is a suspicion of motor disorders such as those just described, esophageal manometry is often useful. Pressures are recorded at various loci by catheters passed through the nose or mouth into the esophagus. While readings are being obtained at various points simultaneously, the patient is given small sips of water to swallow. The recorded pressure changes created by esophageal contractions and variations in sphincter tension can provide a quantitative description of events occurring during swallowing.

A useful test of episodes of acid reflux is 24-hour monitoring of intraesophageal pH. A small pH probe is inserted nasally and affixed 5 cm above the LES. A small battery-powered computer is used for continuous recordings of pH.

■ SUMMARY

1. Swallowing is initiated voluntarily, but, once initiated, it proceeds as an involuntary reflex.
2. Swallowing is accomplished by peristaltic contraction of pharyngeal muscles, during which time the UES relaxes. This is followed by peristaltic contraction of the esophageal musculature, during which time the LES and the orad region of the stomach relax.
3. Peristaltic contraction of the pharyngeal muscles, relaxation of the UES, and peristaltic contraction of the striated muscle of the upper esophagus is regulated by pathways within the central nervous system. Peristaltic contraction of the smooth muscle of the lower esophagus and relaxation of the LES is regulated by pathways within the central nervous system and by pathways within the intrinsic nerves.
4. Contraction of the pharynx and esophagus can be initiated by swallowing (primary peristalsis). Contraction of the esophagus can be initiated by stimulation of receptors within the esophagus (secondary peristalsis).
5. Tonic contraction of the LES between swallows is due to an interplay of excitatory and inhibitory neural and hormonal influences acting on an intrinsic myogenic contraction. During a swallow, intrinsic nerves release a transmitter (perhaps nitric oxide and/or VIP) to cause muscle relaxation.
6. Contraction of the orad stomach is due to an interplay of excitatory and inhibitory neural and hormonal influences acting on an intrinsic myogenic contraction. During a swallow,

the orad stomach relaxes (receptive relaxation) due to activation of inhibitory nerves in the vagus.

■ KEY WORDS AND CONCEPTS

- Oral ingestion of food
- Tongue
- Oral cavity
- Oropharynx
- Nasopharynx
- Glottis
- Larynx
- Peristaltic contraction
- Pharynx
- Upper esophageal sphincter
- Swallowing center
- Esophagus
- Lower esophageal sphincter
- Primary peristalsis
- Secondary peristalsis
- Vagotomy
- Oral portion of the stomach
- Caudad portion of the stomach
- Receptive relaxation
- Achalasia
- Diffuse esophageal spasm
- Acid injury to the esophageal mucosa

■ BIBLIOGRAPHY

Biancani P, Behar J: Esophageal motor function. In Yamada T, editor: *Textbook of gastroenterology*, vol 1, ed 2, Philadelphia, 1995, JB Lippincott.

Conklin JL, Christensen J: Motor functions of the pharynx and esophagus. In Johnson LR, editor: *Physiology of the gastrointestinal tract*, vol 1, ed 3, New York, 1994, Raven Press.

Goyal RK, Paterson WG: Esophageal motility. In Schultz SG, Wood JD, Rauner BB, editors: *Handbook of physiology: the gastrointestinal system*, vol 1, Bethesda, Md, 1989, American Physiological Society.

Roman C, Gonella J: Extrinsic control of digestive tract motility. In Johnson LR, editor: *Physiology of the gastrointestinal tract*, vol 1, ed 2, New York, 1987, Raven Press.

Gastric Emptying

Norman W. Weisbrodt

Motility of the stomach and upper small intestine is organized to accomplish the orderly emptying of contents into the duodenum in the face of variable quantities and compositions of ingested material. Accommodation and temporary storage of ingested material result from receptive relaxation of the orad stomach (discussed in Chapter 3). Emptying, which also requires mixing ingested material with gastric juice and reducing in size any solids that have been swallowed, results from integrated contractions of the orad stomach, the aborad stomach, the pylorus, and the duodenum.

■ ANATOMIC CONSIDERATIONS

Gastric contractions result from activity of smooth muscle cells that are arranged in three layers: an outer longitudinal layer, a middle circular layer, and an inner oblique layer. The **longitudinal layer** is absent on the anterior and posterior surfaces of the stomach. The **circular layer** is the most prominent and is present in all areas of the stomach except the paraesophageal region. The **oblique layer** is the least complete, being formed from two bands of muscle lying on the anterior and posterior surfaces. These two bands meet orally at the gas-troesophageal sphincter and fan out to fuse with the circular muscle layer in the caudad part of the stomach. Both the circular and the longitudinal muscle layers increase in thickness toward the duodenum.

The stomach is richly innervated with both intrinsic and extrinsic nerves. The intrinsic nerves lie in various plexuses, the most prominent being the myenteric plexus that lies in a three-dimensional matrix between the longitudinal and circular muscle layers and throughout the circular muscle layer. The myenteric plexus receives nerve endings from other intrinsic plexuses, as well as from extrinsic nerves. Axons from neurons within the myenteric plexus synapse with the muscle fibers and with glandular cells of the stomach. Extrinsically the stomach is innervated by branches of the vagus nerves and by fibers originating in the celiac plexus of the sympathetic nervous system.

The **pylorus,** or gastroduodenal junction, is characterized by a thickening of the circular muscle layer of the distal antrum. Separating this bundle of muscle from the duodenum is a connective tissue septum; however, some of the longitudinal muscle fibers pass from the antrum to connect with muscle cells of the duodenum. The pylorus is richly innervated with both extrinsic and intrinsic nerves, and nerve endings within the thickened circular muscle layer are abundant. Many of these endings contain neuropeptides, especially enkephalin, and many produce and release nitric oxide.

The anatomy of the proximal duodenum is similar to that of the rest of the intestine and is described in Chapter 5. A significant difference is the larger number of intrinsic nerves present in this area compared with the rest of the small bowel. These may be involved in the regulation of gastric emptying (described below).

■ CONTRACTIONS OF THE ORAD AREA OF THE STOMACH

As detailed in the previous chapter, the predominant motor activity of the orad portion of the stomach is the accommodation of ingested material. During the remainder of the digestive state, a pressure-sensing device placed in the orad stomach detects a resting pressure essentially equal to intraabdominal pressure with superimposed tonic pressure changes. The predominant changes are low amplitude and have a duration of 1 minute or more. The contractions that produce these pressure changes reduce the size of the stomach as the stomach empties. Whether the musculature contracts tonically simply to accommodate the remaining gastric contents, or the muscle contracts to propel material into the caudad stomach, is not known. A consequence of this minimal contractile activity is that little mixing of ingested contents occurs in the orad stomach. Contents often remain in relatively undisturbed layers for an hour or more after eating. Little is known about the regulation of contractions in the orad stomach. Both gastrin and cholecystokinin (CCK) decrease contractions and increase gastric distensibility. However, only the effect of CCK appears to be physiologic.

■ CONTRACTIONS OF THE CAUDAD REGION OF THE STOMACH

Compared with the orad stomach, the caudad region exhibits marked activity. After eating, phasic contractions of varying intensity occur almost continuously. Contractions normally begin in the midstomach and move toward the gastroduodenal junction (Figure 4-1). Thus the primary contractile event is a **peristaltic contraction.** As contractions approach the gastroduodenal junction, they increase in both force and velocity. At any one locus of the human stomach, the duration of each contraction ranges between 2 and 20 seconds, and the maximum frequency is approximately 3 contractions per minute. Between contractions, pressures in the caudad region are near intraabdominal levels.

Contractions of the caudad region of the stomach serve to both mix and propel gastric

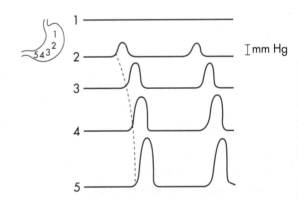

Figure 4-1 ■ Intraluminal pressures recorded from five areas of the stomach. A sensor in the orad region records little phasic activity. Sensors in the caudad region detect peristaltic contractions, which begin in the midportion of the stomach and progress toward the gastroduodenal junction. The contractions increase in force and velocity as they near the junction and repeat at multiple intervals of 12 to 20 seconds. The presence and force of contractions depend on the digestive state of the individual.

contents. Once a contraction begins in the midportion of the stomach, gastric contents are propelled toward the gastroduodenal junction (Figure 4-2, *A*). As the contraction approaches the gastroduodenal junction, some contents are evacuated into the duodenum (Figure 4-2, *B*). However, the increasing velocity of the peristaltic wave as it approaches the junction results in the contraction overtaking the gastric contents. Once this occurs, most of the contents are propelled back into the main body of the stomach (Figure 4-2, *C*). This propulsion back into the stomach has been termed **retropulsion.** Retropulsion causes a thorough mixing of the

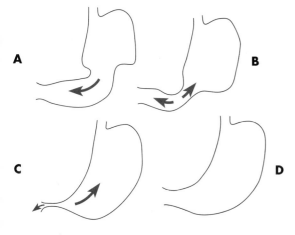

Figure 4-2 ■ Effects that gastric peristaltic contractions have on intraluminal contents. A, The contraction begins in the midregion of the stomach and pushes contents toward the duodenum. B, As the contraction increases in force and velocity, some of the contents are passed over and forced back into the body of the stomach. C, Contraction force and velocity are great enough to cause rapid and almost complete closure of the distal antrum. Before and during this contraction some contents are propelled into the duodenum. However, most are propelled back into the body of the stomach. D, No gross movement of the gastric contents occurs between contractions.

gastric contents and mechanically reduces the size of solid particles.

Contractions of the caudad area of the stomach are controlled by activities of the smooth muscle cells themselves, as well as by nervous and humoral elements. Smooth muscle cells in this area have a membrane potential that fluctuates rhythmically with cyclic depolarizations and repolarizations. These fluctuations are called **slow waves** (also referred to as basic electric rhythm, pacesetter potentials, and control activity). Slow waves have two components: an initial upstroke potential and a secondary plateau potential. In the stomach, slow waves can initiate significant contractions; thus some investigators refer to them as action potentials. However, slow waves are always present, regardless of the presence or absence of contractions. Their frequency is constant and in humans is approximately 3 cycles/min (cpm). If slow waves are recorded from multiple sites between the midstomach and the gastroduodenal junction, they have the same frequency at all sites (Figure 4-3). However, slow waves do not occur simultaneously at all points along the stomach. Rather, a phase lag occurs; thus they seem to pass from an area in the midstomach toward the gastroduodenal junction. This phase lag between slow waves at equidistant points becomes less as the gastroduodenal junction is neared. The frequency and velocity of the peristaltic wave therefore are controlled by the frequency and velocity of spread of the slow wave.

Nervous and humoral factors are not necessary for the presence of slow waves, but they do alter slow wave behavior. Vagotomy disorganizes the slow waves so that the phase lag varies in both duration and direction. The hormone gastrin increases the frequency of gastric slow waves while having little effect on their apparent propagation through the musculature.

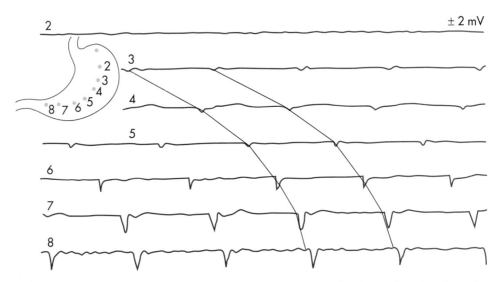

Figure 4-3 ■ Electrical activity of smooth muscle cells of the stomach. Electrodes placed on the serosal surface record no changes from the orad region. In the midregion, however, slow waves occur continuously at intervals of 12 to 20 seconds. Slow waves give the appearance of moving caudad at increasing velocities. Compare this with Figure 4-1. (Adapted from Kelly KA, Code CF, Elveback LR: Patterns of canine gastric electrical activity, *Am J Physiol* 217:461-471, 1969.)

Simultaneous recordings of both electrical and mechanical activities have shown that slow waves initiate significant contractions of the musculature only when the plateau potential exceeds a threshold (Figure 4-4). Once the threshold is exceeded, the greater the amplitude of the plateau, the greater will be the force of contraction. The plateau potential may or may not be accompanied by superimposed rapid oscillations called **spike potentials or spike bursts.** These oscillations also appear to initiate contractions and are seen more frequently in muscle of the caudad antrum. Threshold values for contraction are not reached by every slow wave. Therefore not every slow wave is accompanied by a contraction. If the threshold is reached, it is only during a specific phase of the slow wave cycle. Thus the phasic and peristaltic nature of gastric contractions results from the presence of slow waves.

The amplitude of the plateau potential and therefore the number and force of contractions are markedly influenced by nervous and humoral activities. Vagal nerve transection leads to a decrease in contractions, whereas vagal stimulation increases the frequency and force of contractions. Usually, sympathetic nerve activity depresses contractions. Some hormones, such as gastrin and motilin, increase contractions, whereas others, such as somatostatin, secretin and gastric inhibitory peptide, inhibit them. The physiologic significance of these actions is not known.

■ CONTRACTIONS OF THE GASTRODUODENAL JUNCTION

The question of whether a true sphincter exists between the stomach and duodenum is unsettled. There is a definite difference in the contractile activities of the stomach, on one side, and of the duodenum, on the other. One contracts at a frequency of around 3 cpm, and the other at around 12 cpm. The thickened ring of circular muscle between the two organs appears to behave independently. In humans, some investiga-

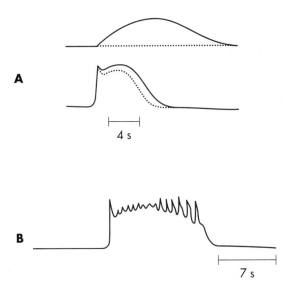

A

4 s

B

7 s

Figure 4-4 ■ **A, Relationship between electrical and mechanical activities of smooth muscle from the caudad region of the stomach. Bottom tracing depicts two slow waves (action potentials) superimposed. Top tracing depicts mechanical events associated with the potential changes. Note that a contraction is initiated only by the slow wave of larger amplitude and longer duration. B, Slow wave potential recorded from distal antrum. Note the oscillations and spike potentials during plateau.** (**A,** Adapted from Szurszewski JH: Mechanism of action of pentagastrin and acetylcholine on the longitudinal muscle of the canine antrum, *J Physiol* 252:335-361, 1975. **B,** Adapted from El-Sharkaway TY, Morgan KG, Szurszewski JH: Intracellular electrical activity of canine and human gastric smooth muscle, *J Physiol* 279:291-307, 1978.)

tors have demonstrated a zone of elevated pressure between the stomach and the duodenum (an indication of sphincteric activity); others, however, have not found such an area. Recent studies have shown that even if a zone of elevated pressure is not found, the pylorus can contract independently, thus altering the resistance to flow between the stomach and duodenum (Figure 4-5). As described below, this can have a large effect on gastric emptying.

■ CONTRACTIONS OF THE PROXIMAL DUODENUM

Duodenal contractions are mostly phasic. Although their maximum frequency can be around 12 per minute in the digestive state, they seldom occur in a continuous manner. Rather, single isolated or small groups of contractions, separated by intervals of no contractions, are the norm. Also, duodenal contractions are not always peristaltic. As discussed in Chapter 5, most contractions of the small intestine are of the segmenting type. Thus depending upon their number and pattern, duodenal contractions either impede or facilitate the emptying of contents from the stomach.

■ REGULATION OF GASTRIC EMPTYING

Immediately after ingestion of a meal the stomach may contain over a liter of material, which then takes several hours to leave the stomach and empty into the small intestine. Gastric emptying is accomplished by coordinated contractile activity of the stomach, pylorus, and proximal small intestine (Figure 4-6). Emptying appears to be regulated in a manner that allows for optimal intestinal digestion and absorption of foodstuffs (Figure 4-7). Solids empty only after a lag period during which time they are reduced in size by retropulsive activity of the caudad stomach. Liquids begin to empty almost immediately. The rate of emptying of both solids and liquids depends upon their chemical compositions. Materials that are high in lipids or H^+, or that deviate markedly from isotonicity, all empty at a slower rate than do near isotonic saline solutions.

Regulation results from the presence of receptors that lie in the upper small bowel. These receptors appear to respond to the physical properties (such as osmotic pressure) and chemical composition (H^+, lipids) of the chyme. As chyme empties from the stomach, **intestinal receptors** are activated. Receptor activation in turn results in an inhibition of emptying through pathways that are incompletely understood.

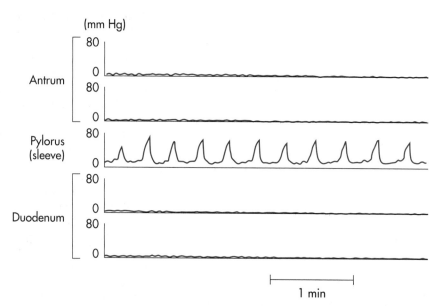

Figure 4-5 ■ Intraluminal pressures recorded from two areas of the stomach (*antrum*), the pylorus, and two areas of the proximal duodenum during the intraduodenal infusion of lipid. Note the regular isolated contractions, and the elevated pressures (*0* indicates atmospheric pressure in each tracing) between contractions, in the pylorus. This activity is occurring at a time when there are no contractions present in the stomach and duodenum. (Adapted from Heddle R, Dent J, Read NW, Houghton LA: Antropyloroduodenal motor responses to intraduodenal lipid infusion in healthy volunteers, *Am J Physiol* 254:G671-G679, 1988.)

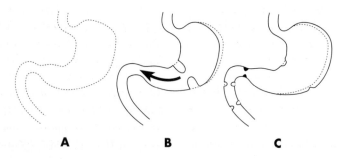

Figure 4-6 ■ Regulation of gastric emptying. A, Hypothetical conditions immediately after the rapid ingestion of a meal and before the onset of any contractile activity. This outline is superimposed in B and C to illustrate changes. B, Conditions favoring emptying are increased tone of the orad region of the stomach, forceful peristaltic contractions of the caudad region of the stomach, relaxation of the pylorus, and absence of segmenting contractions of the duodenum. As nutrients emptied from the stomach are further digested and absorbed in the small intestine, they excite receptors located in the intestinal mucosa. Activation of these receptors results in C: relaxation of the orad region of the stomach, a decrease in the number and force of contractions of the caudad region of the stomach, contraction of the pylorus, and an increase in segmenting contractions of the duodenum. This results in a slowing of gastric emptying.

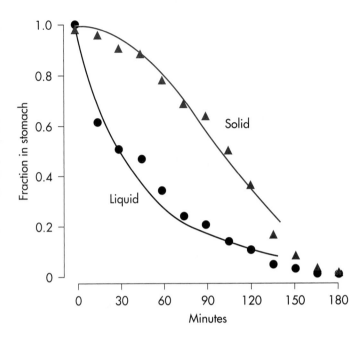

Figure 4-7 ■ **Solid and liquid components of a meal were labeled so that their emptying from the stomach could be followed over time after ingestion of the meal. As indicated by the sharp decrease in the fraction remaining in the stomach, the liquid component began to empty almost immediately, and it emptied more rapidly. On the other hand, there was a lag time before the emptying of the label attached to the solid component, and this label emptied more slowly. This slower emptying was due to the fact that the solid component had to be reduced to small particles before being emptied into the duodenum.** (Adapted from Camilleri M, Malagelada JR, Brown ML, Becker G: Relation between antral motility and gastric emptying of solids and liquids in humans, *Am J Physiol* 249:G580-G585, 1985.)

Many of the substances that inhibit gastric emptying also release one or more **gastrointestinal (GI) hormones;** and many of the hormones slow gastric emptying when injected. Thus it is tempting to speculate that foodstuffs inhibit emptying by releasing hormones. However, such a causal relationship has been hard to establish. It is just as likely that these receptors regulate emptying through neural mechanisms.

Regulation of gastric emptying is brought about by alterations in motility of the stomach, gastroduodenal junction, and duodenum. Decreases in distensibility of the orad stomach, increases in the force of peristaltic contractions of the caudad stomach, increases in diameter and inhibition of contractions of the pylorus, and inhibition of segmenting contractions of the proximal duodenum all lead to an increase in the rate of gastric emptying. Upon activation of the duodenal receptors just mentioned, one or more of these contractile activities of the stomach and the duodenum are reversed to slow emptying (Figure 4-6).

The pattern of motility of the gastroduodenal area changes after the nutrient components of the meal have been digested and absorbed. Any large particles of undigested residue that remain in the stomach are emptied by a burst of peristaltic contractions as part of the migrating motor complex (MMC) (Figure 4-8). During this short burst, powerful contractions begin in the previously inactive orad region and sweep the entire length of the stomach. The pylorus dilates and the duodenum relaxes during each sweep, so that the resistance to emptying is minimal. Then **duodenal contractions** sweep the contents onward as discussed in Chapter 5. After a burst of activity, the region remains relaxed for an hour or more. Then intermittent contractions begin and lead to another burst. This cycle repeats every 90 minutes or so until ingestion of the next meal. Premature bursts can be initiated by injection of the hormone motilin and by drugs (e.g., erythromycin) thought to act on motilin receptors.

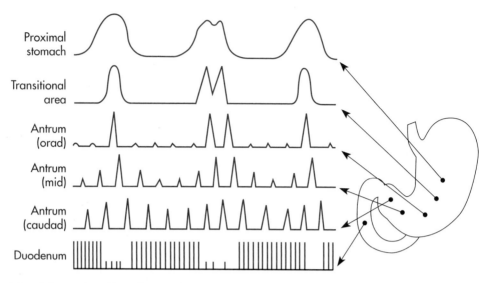

Figure 4-8 ■ Schematic of intraluminal pressures recorded from the stomach and proximal duodenum during an active phase of an MMC. Note that phasic contractions begin in the orad region of the stomach and propagate over the caudad region. As contractions of the caudad region approach the gastroduodenal junction, the pylorus relaxes (not shown) and duodenal contractions are momentarily inhibited. This allows contents to be swept into the duodenum. Contents are then propelled toward the colon as described in Chapter 5. (Adapted from Malagelada J-R, Azpiroz F: Determinants of gastric emptying and transit in the small intestine. In Schultz SG, Wood JD, Rauner BB, editors: *The gastrointestinal system*, vol 1, Bethesda, Md, 1989, American Physiological Society, p 909.)

■ CLINICAL APPLICATIONS

Disorders of gastric motility are generally manifested by a rate of gastric emptying that is either too slow or too fast. This may reflect an abnormality in one or all of the major motor functions of the stomach. When the stomach fails to empty properly, nausea, loss of appetite, and early satiety are experienced, and often gastric contents may be vomited. The most common form of impaired emptying results from obstruction at the gastric outlet. Examples are gastric cancer and peptic ulcer disease. In the latter, inflammation and scarring associated with the ulcer may actually occlude the gastric lumen at the pylorus. Impaired emptying also can be caused by the absence or disorganization of motor events in the

caudad stomach. These phenomena occur in a variety of metabolic disorders, such as diabetes mellitus and potassium depletion.

Vagus nerve section **(vagotomy)** invariably leads to delay of gastric emptying of solids. Consequently vagotomy (to decrease acid secretion in peptic ulcer disease) is coupled with alterations of the pylorus **(pyloroplasty)** or creation of a new gastric outlet **(gastroenterostomy)** in an attempt to avoid this complication. After such an operation, emptying of liquids is generally accelerated; but even with alteration of the gastric outlet, emptying of solids still may be slowed. The majority of patients undergoing this type of surgery experience no other symptoms. However, some may experience diarrhea, sweating, palpitations, cramps, and a variety of other unpleasant symptoms, which result from changes in gastric emptying.

It is speculated that motility abnormalities may underlie or contribute to other diseases of the upper GI tract. For example, gastric emptying is accelerated in patients with duodenal ulcer. This may enhance the delivery of gastric acid to the duodenum, perhaps overwhelming the ability of the duodenal mucosa to defend itself against injury. Alternatively, in patients with gastric ulcer, gastric emptying appears to be slowed. This may create a situation in which the stomach is more susceptible to injury.

■ CLINICAL TESTS

For a variety of reasons, motor events in the stomach do not lend themselves to clinical assessment with techniques such as those used in the esophagus. Therefore evaluation of gastric motility is often limited to qualitative observations of gastric emptying provided by x-ray and fluoroscopic evaluation of a barium-filled stomach. Occasionally aspiration of the stomach at a specific interval after installation of an isotonic saline solution will give information regarding gastric emptying. One quantitative test that is gaining acceptance is γ-scintigraphy. For this test, radiolabeled liquid and/or solid food is ingested, and gamma cameras are used to scan the stomach at various times afterward. The fraction of material remaining in the stomach is then plotted as a function of time (Figure 4-7).

■ SUMMARY

1. Contractile activity of the orad stomach varies with the digestive state. After the orad region has accommodated a meal, it exhibits low-amplitude long-lasting contractions as the meal empties. After the meal has been digested and absorbed, the orad stomach undergoes periodic bursts of high-amplitude contractions as part of the MMC.

2. Contractions of the aborad stomach are mostly peristaltic, beginning in the midstomach and progressing toward the duodenum. During emptying of a meal, contractions are of variable amplitude and are more or less continuous at a frequency of about 3 per minute. During the interdigestive period, forceful peristaltic contractions are grouped into periodic bursts as part of the MMC.

3. Gastric emptying is highly regulated and involves feedback inhibition from receptors located in the upper small intestine. Receptors are stimulated by osmotic pressure, hydrogen ions, and fatty acids. Stimulation results in patterns of motility that slow emptying: decreased tonic contraction of the orad stomach, decreased force and number of contractions of the aborad stomach, increased tone and phasic contractions of the pylorus, and increased segmenting contractions of the upper duodenum.

4. Rhythmic membrane depolarizations and repolarizations called slow waves occur in smooth muscle cells of the aborad stomach. They are omnipresent occurring at a frequency of about 3 per minute. Each depolarization appears to be initiated first in the midstomach and then to propagate toward the pylorus. Slow waves appear to set the timing and the peristaltic nature of contractions; however, not every slow wave initiates a contraction. Those that do are of large amplitude and may exhibit superimposed spike potentials.

5. Vagotomy results in a decrease in number and force of contractions of the aborad stomach and a decrease in gastric emptying of solids. Motilin induces contractions that are part of the gastric phase of the MMC.

■ KEY WORDS AND CONCEPTS

- Longitudinal muscle layer of the stomach
- Circular muscle layer of the stomach
- Oblique layer of the stomach
- Pylorus
- Peristaltic contraction
- Retropulsion
- Slow waves
- Spike potentials or spike bursts
- Intestinal receptors
- Gastrointestinal hormones
- Duodenal contractions
- Vagotomy
- Pyloroplasty
- Gastroenterostomy

■ BIBLIOGRAPHY

Ehrlein HJ, Akkermans LMA: Gastric emptying. In Akkermans LMA, Johnson AG, Read NW, editors: *Gastric and gastroduodenal motility*, New York, 1984, Praeger.

Hunt JN, Knox MT: Regulation of gastric emptying. In Code CF, editor: *Handbook of physiology*, vol 4, Baltimore, 1968, Williams & Wilkins.

Malagelada J-R, Azpiroz F: Determinants of gastric emptying and transit in the small intestine. In Schultz SG, Wood JD, Rauner BB, editors: *Handbook of physiology: the gastrointestinal system*, Bethesda, Md, 1989, American Physiological Society.

Mayer EA: The physiology of gastric storage and emptying. In Johnson LR, editor: *Physiology of the gastrointestinal tract*, vol 1, ed 3, New York, 1994, Raven Press.

Motility of the Small Intestine

Norman W. Weisbrodt

Motility of the small intestine is organized to optimize the processes of digestion and absorption of nutrients and the aboral propulsion of undigested material. Thus contractions perform at least three functions: (1) mixing of ingested foodstuffs with digestive secretions and enzymes; (2) circulation of all intestinal contents to facilitate contact with the intestinal mucosa; and (3) net propulsion of the intestinal contents in an aboral direction.

■ ANATOMIC CONSIDERATIONS

Contractions of the small intestine are effected by activities of two layers of smooth muscle cells: an **outer layer** with the long axis of the cells arranged longitudinally and an **inner layer** with the long axis of the cells arranged circularly. In general the circular muscle layer is thicker, and both layers are more abundant in the proximal intestine, decreasing in thickness distally to the level of the ileocecal junction.

The small intestine is richly innervated by elements of the autonomic nervous system. Within the wall of the intestine itself lie neurons, nerve endings, and receptors of the enteric nervous system. (See Figure 2-2.) These neural elements tend to be concentrated in several plexuses. The most

prominent, the **myenteric or Auerbach plexus,** lies between the circular and longitudinal layers of smooth muscle cells. Plexal neurons receive input from other neurons within the plexus, from receptors located in the mucosa and muscle walls, and from the central nervous system by way of the parasympathetic and sympathetic nerve trunks. Plexal neurons provide integrated output to smooth muscle cells of both muscle layers, to epithelial cells, and perhaps to endocrine and immune cells. Many neurotransmitters are present in the enteric nervous system including acetylcholine, norepinephrine, vasoactive intestinal peptide, enkephalin, and other peptides. Furthermore, many nerves express nitric oxide synthase activity.

Extrinsic innervation is supplied by the vagus nerve and by nerve fibers from the celiac and superior mesenteric ganglia. (See Figure 2-1.) Many of the fibers within the vagus are preganglionic, whereas many from the abdominal ganglia are postganglionic. Some of the fibers within the vagus are cholinergic, whereas some from the abdominal plexuses are adrenergic. In addition, nerves that contain somatostatin, substance P, cholecystokinin, enkephalin, neuropeptide Y, and other transmitters have been identified in afferent and efferent vagal and splanchnic nerves. The exact pathways and physiologic roles of these nerves are being elucidated.

■ TYPES OF CONTRACTIONS

Between contractions, pressures within the lumen of the small intestine approximately equal intraabdominal pressure. When the musculature contracts, the lumen is occluded partially or totally, and pressure increases. Most contractions are local events and involve only 1 to 4 cm of bowel at a time. The contractions usually produce intraluminal pressure waves that appear as nearly symmetrical peaks of uniform shape (Figure 5-1). In the human upper small bowel, contractions occur at any one site at multiple intervals of 5 seconds (Figure 5-2).

Occasionally other types of pressure waves can be recorded. One such type consists of an el-

evated baseline pressure that lasts from 10 seconds to 8 minutes. This wave seldom occurs alone, usually being accompanied by superimposed phasic changes in pressure.

The effect that any contraction has on intestinal contents depends upon the state of the musculature above and below the point of the contraction. If a contraction is not coordinated with activity above and below, intestinal contents are displaced both proximally and distally during the contraction and may flow back during the period of relaxation. This would serve to mix and locally circulate the contents (Figure 5-3, *A*). Such contractions appear to divide the bowel into segments, which accounts for the name **segmentation** given to this process. If, however, the contractions at adjacent sites occur in a proximal-to-distal sequence, aboral propulsion will result.

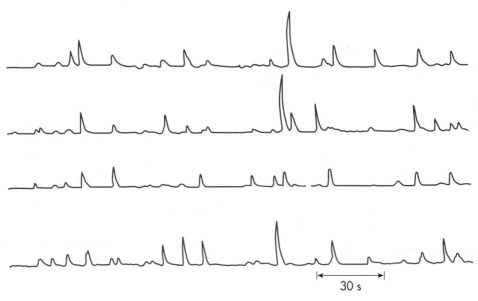

Figure 5-1 ■ Intraluminal pressure changes recorded from the duodenum of a conscious human. Sensors placed 1 cm apart record changes in pressure that are phasic, lasting 4 to 5 seconds. Note that a rather large contraction can take place at one site while nothing is recorded 1 cm away on either side.

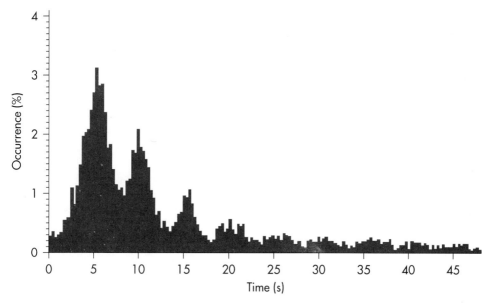

Figure 5-2 ■ Frequency distribution of 7572 contractions recorded at one site in the human small intestine. Note that the contractions are most frequent at multiples of 5 seconds, which is the approximate interval between slow waves in this region. (From Christensen J, Glover JR, Macagno EO, Singerman RB, Weisbrodt NW: Statistics of contractions at a point in the human duodenum, *Am J Physiol* 221:1818-1823, 1971.)

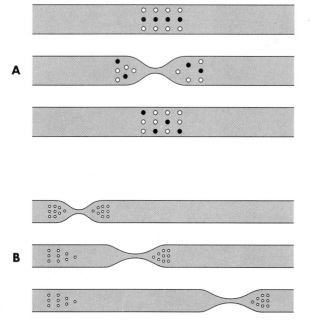

Figure 5-3 ■ The influence of contractions on contents within a region of intestine. Each panel depicts the region at three consecutive points in time. A, A contraction that is neither preceded nor followed by other contractions serves to mix and locally circulate the intestinal contents. B, Contractions that have an orad-to-aborad sequence *(left to right)* serve to propel contents in a net aboral direction.

The small intestine also is capable of eliciting a highly coordinated contractile response that is propulsive in function. When an area of bowel is stimulated (e.g., by placement of a solid bolus of material in the lumen), the bowel responds with contraction orad and relaxation aborad to the point of stimulation. These events tend to move the material in an aboral direction (Figure 5-3, *B*), and if they occur sequentially they can propel a bolus the entire length of the gut in a short time. This peristaltic response, first described by Bayliss and Starling, is known as the **law of the intestines.** Often it is invoked to explain how material normally is propelled through the small bowel. Recently, however, its importance in healthy individuals has been downgraded. Peristalsis involving long segments of intestine is seldom seen in normal individuals, although short (1 to 4 cm) peristaltic contractions have been described.

■ PATTERNS OF CONTRACTIONS

Not only are there differences in individual contractions of the intestine, there are also different patterns of contractions. In the fasting human, contractions do not occur evenly over time. Rather, at each locus there are cycles comprised of phases of no or few contractions, followed by a phase of intense contractions that ends abruptly (Figure 5-4). The duration of each cycle is the same at adjacent loci of the bowel; however, the 5- to 10-minute phase of intense contractions does not occur simultaneously at all loci. Instead, this phase appears to migrate aborally, taking approximately 1.5 hours to sweep from the duodenum through the ileum. The characteristics of this pattern have earned it the title of **migrating motor complex** (MMC). This complex actually begins in the stomach. (See Chapter 4.) Its functions

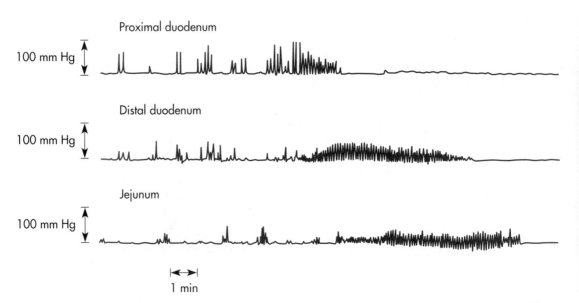

Figure 5-4 ■ Contractions at three loci in the small bowel. Note that at each locus, phases of no or intermittent contractions are followed by a phase of continuous contractions that ends abruptly. Also note that the phase of continuous contractions appears to migrate aborally along the bowel. Such a pattern is called the MMC. (From Rees WD, Malagelada JR, Miller H: Human interdigestive and postprandial gastrointestinal motor and gastrointestinal hormone patterns, *Dig Dis Sci* 27:321-329, 1982.)

appear to be to sweep undigested contents from the stomach, through the small intestine, and into the colon; and to maintain low bacterial counts in the upper intestine. MMCs cycle at intervals of about every 1.5 hours (Figure 5-5) as long as the individual is fasting.

In a nonfasting individual, contractions are spread more uniformly over time. In the upper human small bowel, contractions are present 14% to 34% of the recorded time, with the most common pattern being one to three sequential contractions separated by periods of 5, 10, 15, or 20 seconds. These contractions are of varying intensity, with none being as forceful as the intense contractions that occur during the MMC.

Contractions of the intestine are controlled by activities of the smooth muscle cells themselves, as well as by nerves and humoral substances. As in the stomach, smooth muscle cells in the small intestine have a membrane potential that fluctuates rhythmically with cyclic depolarizations and repolarizations of 5 to 15 mV (Figure 5-6). This **slow wave activity** (or basic electrical rhythm) is always present whether contractions are occurring or not. At any one site in the intestine, slow wave frequency is constant. Frequency, however, is not the same at all levels of the bowel. There is a decrease in frequency toward the ileocecal junction. In humans the frequency decreases from a mean of about 12 cycles/min (cpm) in the duodenum to a mean of about 8 cpm in the terminal ileum. The decrease is not linear because frequency is constant throughout the duodenum and for about 10 cm into the jejunum. Beyond that point frequency declines more or less linearly.

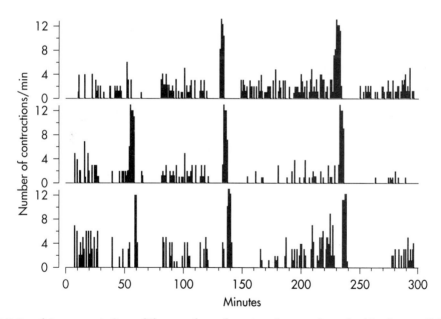

Figure 5-5 ■ Graphic presentation of the number of contractions at three loci in the small bowel. The number of contractions during each minute of the recording was counted and plotted against the time of recording. The resulting histogram indicates cycles of activity at each locus. Note that MMCs recur at each locus at intervals of about 100 minutes and that the phases of intense contractions appear to migrate aborally. (From Vantrappen G, Janssens J: The interdigestive motor complex of normal subjects and patients with bacterial overgrowth of the small intestine, *J Clin Invest* 59:1158-1166, 1977.)

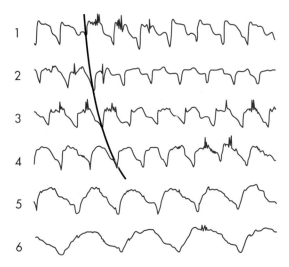

Figure 5-6 ▪ Slow waves and spike potentials from multiple sites in the small intestine. Tracings 1 to 6 illustrate activity from progressively distal areas. Solid line connecting the slow waves in tracings 1 to 4 denotes the apparent propagation in the region of a slow wave frequency plateau. Tracings 5 and 6 show decreases in slow wave frequency at more distal areas. The rapid transients that occur on the peaks of some of the slow waves represent spike potentials.

Although slow wave frequency is identical over the proximal small intestine, slow waves do not occur simultaneously at all points. Multiple electrodes detect a proximal-to-distal phase lag that simulates a propagated signal (Figure 5-6).

In the small intestine, slow waves themselves do not initiate forceful contractions. Contractions are initiated by a second electrical event, often referred to as spike potential activity. **Spike potentials** are rapid depolarizations of the smooth muscle cell membrane that occur only during the depolarization phase of the slow wave. Because spike potentials are restricted to only one phase of the slow wave cycle, the contractions they initiate are phasic in nature. The muscle relaxes during the repolarization phase of the slow wave cycle.

During periods of time when every slow wave is accompanied by spike potentials, the intestine at any site contracts at the same frequency as the slow wave frequency at that site. Thus slow wave frequency sets the maximum frequency of contractions at any one site. Also, since a gradient exists in the slow wave frequency along the small bowel, there is a gradient in the maximal frequency of contractions. For most of the time, however, spike potentials do not accompany every slow wave. During these periods, contractions at any one site occur at multiples of the slow wave interval. Thus it is no coincidence that in the human proximal bowel, slow waves occur every 5 seconds and contractions occur at multiple intervals of 5 seconds.

Although slow waves at adjacent sites along the bowel are always present and are temporally related, the occurrence of spike potentials often is localized. Thus sites 1 to 2 cm on either side of an area exhibiting slow waves with spike potentials may exhibit slow waves only. When this is the situation, segmenting contractions occur. On the other hand, when the occurrence of spike potentials is not localized, slow waves do influence the spatial relationships of contractions at adjacent sites. The phase lag in occurrence of slow waves at adjacent sites imposes a phase lag in the occurrence of contractions at adjacent sites. Thus it is not surprising to learn that a peristaltic contraction moves at the same velocity as the apparent velocity of the slow wave.

As explained above, not every slow wave is accompanied by spike potentials and muscle contraction. Occurrence of spike potentials and contractions is regulated by nervous activity and by circulating and locally released chemical agents. There are a number of reflexes that depend upon the intrinsic neurons, the extrinsic neurons, or both. The **peristaltic reflex** (law of the intestines) described previously depends on an intact enteric nervous system. Application of neural blocking agents will abolish or greatly reduce this reflex. Another reflex, the **intestino-intestinal reflex,** depends upon extrinsic neural connections. If an area of the bowel is grossly distended, contractile activity in the rest of the bowel is inhibited. Sectioning of the extrinsic nerves abolishes this reflex. Additionally, it is well known that changes in the emotional state of an individual can induce alterations in small bowel motility. Thus the small bowel is under the influence of higher centers of the nervous system.

In addition to neural control, many circulating and endogenously released chemicals alter intestinal motility. Epinephrine released from the adrenal glands tends to inhibit contractions. Serotonin, which is contained in large quantities within the small intestine, stimulates contractions, as do certain of the prostaglandins. Several hormones also alter intestinal motility. Gastrin, cholecystokinin (CCK), motilin, and insulin tend to stimulate contractions, whereas secretin and glucagon tend to inhibit them. The exact role of these chemical agents in the regulation of motility is yet to be clarified.

The presence of a characteristic pattern of contractions during fasting (the MMC) indicates complex controlling mechanisms. The hormone motilin may be involved in regulating MMC cycle length. Plasma levels of motilin fluctuate with the same periodicity as the phase of intense duodenal contractions, and exogenously administered motilin will initiate a premature MMC. Enteric nerves are also involved since their disruption alters MMC initiation and migration. Extrinsic nerves do not seem to be required. Segments of intestine that have been extrinsically denervated still exhibit MMCs. However, extrinsic neural activity can modify characteristics of the MMC.

Feeding abolishes MMCs and institutes a pattern of more or less continuous contractions of varying amplitude. The change in pattern with feeding probably is brought about by hormones such as gastrin and CCK, which are released during feeding, and by neural mechanisms.

■ CLINICAL APPLICATION

Primary disorders of small intestine motility probably are rare. The small intestine may be involved in certain general disorders of smooth muscle of the gastrointestinal and urinary tracts. The cause of these disorders is unknown, but in some patients there may be a genetic basis. When the disorder is clinically apparent, the patient appears to have episodes of intestinal obstruction; however, the problem seems to involve failure of propulsive motility rather than obstruction. Thus the name **idiopathic pseudoobstruction** has been coined. In some patients with this syndrome, the smooth muscle cells are involved. In others, histologic studies show changes in enteric nerves rather than in smooth muscle.

Altered small intestinal motility resulting in delayed transit frequently accompanies a variety of diseases and clinical situations. Perhaps the most common is the transient ileus or apparent paralysis of the small intestine sometimes seen after abdominal surgery. However, intraabdominal inflammation (pancreatitis, appendicitis, abscess, etc.) may produce a similar picture. Systemic diseases such as diabetes mellitus and amyloidosis, metabolic alterations such as potassium depletion, and administration of drugs, particularly anticholinergics, all may have an adverse effect on intestinal transit. Mixing is likely impaired as well, although this is less clinically apparent.

Alternatively, rapid intestinal transit is seen in certain malabsorptive states induced by infectious agents, allergic reaction, and various pharmacologic agents. In these conditions both motility and absorption are affected. In most disease states it is not clear whether changes in motility are primary (caused by the disease) or secondary (caused by the presence of unabsorbed or secreted material). The types and patterns of contractions that underlie these conditions are the subject of current investigation.

■ CLINICAL TESTS

Because of the inaccessibility of the small intestine, direct measurement of contractions or electrical activity is difficult and, as yet, not used routinely. Often auscultation to detect "sounds" is used to assess bowel activity. In addition, observing the movement of barium can yield some information on transit time through the small bowel. Unfortunately, however, the wide range of normal values for intestinal transit makes it difficult to utilize transit time as a diagnostic tool unless transit is markedly altered.

■ SUMMARY

1. Movement of contents within the intestinal lumen depends upon the type of contraction. Segmenting contractions cause mixing and local circulation of contents. Peristaltic contractions cause net aboral transit.
2. During digestion of a meal, most contractions are of the segmenting type with short peristaltic contractions occurring randomly. During interdigestive periods, bursts of intense peristaltic contractions envelop each region of the intestine about every 90 minutes. Each burst appears to begin in the stomach and to migrate aborally along the intestine such that it reaches the terminal ileum in about 90 minutes. This activity is called the migrating motor complex or MMC.
3. Intestinal slow waves are cyclic depolarizations and repolarizations of muscle cell membranes. At any locus of the intestine, slow waves are present at a constant frequency (e.g., around 12 per minute in the duodenum and 8 per minute in the ileum). At adjacent loci, slow waves appear to propagate aborally.
4. Spike potentials are rapid fluctuations in membrane potential that are superimposed on the depolarization phase of the slow wave. They, not the slow waves themselves, initiate contractions of the muscle. Spike potentials do not accompany every slow wave. Their presence and pattern depend upon the digestive state of the animal and on neural and humoral activities.
5. Enteric nerves coordinate both the type and patterns of contraction. The phase of intense contractions of the MMC in the upper intestine may be initiated by the release of motilin. The conversion of the MMC pattern to the digestive pattern may in part be due to the release of hormones such as gastrin and CCK.

■ KEY WORDS AND CONCEPTS

- Outer muscle layer of the small intestine
- Inner muscle layer of the small intestine
- Myenteric or Auerbach plexus
- Segmentation
- Law of the intestines
- Migrating motor complex
- Slow wave activity
- Spike potentials
- Peristaltic reflex
- Intestino-intestinal reflex
- Idiopathic pseudoobstruction

■ BIBLIOGRAPHY

Hasler WL: Motility of the small intestine. In Yamada T, editor: *Textbook of gastroenterology,* vol 1, ed 2, Philadelphia, 1995, JB Lippincott.

Weisbrodt NW: Motility of the small intestine. In Johnson LR, editor: *Physiology of the gastrointestinal tract,* New York, 1987, Raven Press.

Wingate DL: Backward and forward with the migrating complex, *Dig Dis Sci* 26:641-666, 1981.

Motility of the Large Intestine

Norman W. Weisbrodt

C ontractions of the large intestine are organized to allow for optimum absorption of water and electrolytes, net aboral movement of contents, and the storage and orderly evacuation of feces.

■ ANATOMIC CONSIDERATIONS

Anatomically the human large intestine is divided into the **cecum;** the **ascending, transverse, descending, and sigmoid colon;** the **rectum;** and the **anal canal.** The muscular layers of the large intestine are composed of both longitudinally and circularly arranged fibers. Longitudinal fibers are concentrated into three flat bands called the **taeniae coli.** These run from the cecum to the rectum, where the fibers fan out to form a more continuous longitudinal coat. The circular layer of muscle fibers is continuous from the cecum to the anal canal, where it increases in thickness to form the internal anal sphincter. Overlapping and slightly distal to the internal anal sphincter are layers of striated muscle. These striated muscle bundles make up the **external anal sphincter.**

In humans the external features of the large intestine differ from those of the small intestine. In addition to the presence of taeniae coli, the colon appears to be divided into segments called **haustra or haustrations** (Figure 6-1). Haustra are probably the result of structural and functional properties of the colon. Points of concentration of muscular tissue and mucosal foldings can be found in colons examined postmortem. Also, haustra are more prominent in areas of the colon that possess taeniae coli. Haustra are not fixed, however. Segmental colonic contractions appear, disappear, and re-form at another locus. Thus haustral formation also has a dynamic component because of the contractile activity of colonic musculature.

The large intestine, like other areas of the bowel, is innervated by the autonomic nervous system (ANS). The enteric system consists partly of many nerve cell bodies and endings that lie between the circular and longitudinal muscle coats. In areas of the large intestine with taeniae, this myenteric plexus is concentrated beneath them. Cells of the myenteric plexus receive input from a variety of receptors within the intestine, as well as by way of the extrinsic nerves. Axons from these cells innervate the muscle layers. Extrinsic innervation to the large intestine comes from both parasympathetic and sympathetic branches of the ANS. There are two pathways of

51

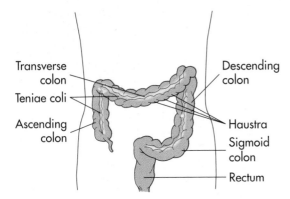

Transverse colon

Teniae coli

Ascending colon

Descending colon

Haustra

Sigmoid colon

Rectum

Figure 6-1 ■ **Anatomy of the colon. The colon is short and large in diameter when compared with the small intestine.   The longitudinal smooth muscle is concentrated into three bands *(taeniae coli)* in all regions except the rectum. Note that all regions except the rectum possess haustra. The exact cause of haustration is not known. They are formed partly by contractions of the circular muscle; however, because they are still present after death, some investigators believe they have a permanent structural basis.**

parasympathetic innervation: the cecum and the ascending and transverse portions of the colon are innervated by the vagus nerve; the descending and sigmoid areas of the colon and the rectum are innervated by pelvic nerves from the sacral region of the spinal cord. The pelvic nerves enter the colon near the rectosigmoid junction and project orally and aborally within the plane of the myenteric plexus. These projections, called **shunt fascicles,** innervate myenteric nerves en route. The vagus and pelvic nerves consist primarily of preganglionic efferent fibers and many afferent fibers. The efferent fibers supposedly synapse with the nerve cell bodies of the myenteric and other intrinsic plexuses. The proximal regions of the large intestine are sympathetically innervated by fibers that come from the superior mesenteric ganglion. More distal regions receive input from the inferior mesenteric ganglion. The distal rectum

and anal canal are innervated by sympathetic fibers from the hypogastric plexus. Most of the sympathetic fibers are postganglionic efferent and afferent fibers. The external anal sphincter, a striated muscle, is innervated by the somatic pudendal nerves.

As in other regions of the gut, a number of diverse chemicals serve as mediators at presynaptic and postsynaptic junctions within the autonomic innervation to the large intestine. Acetylcholine (ACh) and tachykinins such as substance P serve as major excitatory mediators, and nitric oxide, vasoactive intestinal peptide, and possibly adenosine triphosphate serve as major inhibitory mediators. Transmission between the pudendal nerves and the external anal sphincter is mediated by ACh.

■ CONTRACTIONS OF THE CECUM AND ASCENDING COLON

Flow of contents from the small intestine into the large intestine is intermittent and regulated partly by a sphincteric mechanism at the **ileocecal junction.** A sensor placed in the junction records pressures that are several millimeters of mercury greater than those in the ileum or colon. The pressure, however, is not constant, for the sphincter relaxes periodically; during this time ileal contractions propel contents into the large intestine (Figure 6-2, *A*). Once material reaches the proximal large intestine, it is acted on by a wide variety of contractions. The majority of these are segmental in nature, with durations of 12 to 60 seconds. The pressures generated by these contractions vary in amplitude between about 10 and 50 mm Hg. It is believed that these contractions are partly responsible for the haustrations seen in the colon. At adjacent sites contractions usually occur independently. Thus they slowly move the contents back and forth, mixing and exposing them to the mucosa for absorption of water and electrolytes. In addition to pressure changes caused by segmental

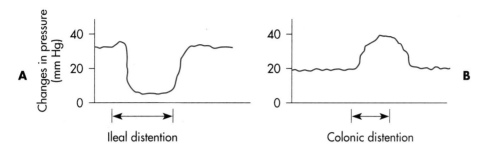

Figure 6-2 ■ Intraluminal pressures recorded at the level of the ileocecal sphincter. Note that a resting pressure of 20 to 40 mm Hg exists. A, Distention of the ileum causes sphincteric relaxation and thus allows flow of contents from the ileum into the colon. B, Distention of the colon, on the other hand, causes contraction of the sphincter to prevent passage of contents from the colon to the ileum. (From Cohen S, Harris LD, Levitan R: Manometric characteristics of the human ileocecal junctional zone, *Gastroenterology* 54:72-75, 1968.)

contractions, a large variety of other pressure waves has been recorded. Attempts to classify these have been made, but the degree of overlap of pressure profiles makes classification difficult.

Occasionally segmental contractions are organized in an orad-to-aboral direction; thus propulsion over short distances takes place. Most propulsion, however, occurs during a characteristic sequence termed **mass movement.** Segmental activity suddenly ceases, and along with its disappearance there is a loss of haustrations. The colon then undergoes a contraction that sweeps intraluminal contents in an aboral direction (Figure 6-3, *A* to *C*). Following the mass movement, haustrations and phasic contractions return (Figure 6-3, *D*). Mass movements are infrequent in healthy people and are estimated to occur only 1 to 3 times daily. Because they are such infrequent events, they have not been studied in any great detail in normal individuals.

■ CONTRACTIONS OF THE DESCENDING AND SIGMOID COLON

By the time material reaches the descending and sigmoid colon, it has changed from a liquid to a semisolid state. Although there is less absorption of water and electrolytes from these portions of the colon, motility studies have demonstrated that contractions of the segmenting type are more frequent here than in the ascending and transverse colon. These segmenting contractions do not result in propulsion. On the contrary, they offer resistance and thus retard the flow of contents from more proximal regions into the rectum. Propulsion into and through these areas also probably occurs during mass movements. Here, too, there is loss of segmental activity and the haustrations that precede transport (Figure 6-3, *E* and *F*). Thus material that enters these regions during a mass movement is acted on to further reduce its liquid content and is then propelled into the rectum during a subsequent mass movement.

■ MOTILITY OF THE RECTUM AND ANAL CANAL

The rectum is usually empty or nearly so. Although few contents are present, contractions do occur in this region. In fact, the upper regions of the rectum contract segmentally more frequently than does the sigmoid colon. This activity tends to retard the flow of contents into the rectum. When the rectum fills it does so intermittently. During a mass movement or during an aborally directed sequence of segmental contractions of the sigmoid colon, some material passes into the rectum.

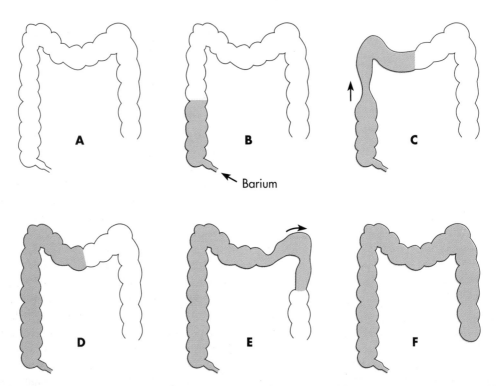

Figure 6-3 ■ Two mass movements. A, Appearance of the colon before the entry of barium sulfate. B, As the barium enters from the ileum, it is acted on by haustral contractions. C, As more barium enters a portion is swept into and through an area of the colon that has lost its haustral markings. D, The barium is acted on by the haustral contractions that have returned. E, A second mass movement propels the barium into and through areas of the transverse and descending colon. F, Haustrations again return. Most of the movement of feces through the colon is accomplished by this type of contraction.

Normally the anal canal is closed because of contraction of the internal anal sphincter. When the rectum is distended by fecal material, however, the internal sphincter relaxes as part of the **rectosphincteric reflex** (Figure 6-4). Rectal distention also elicits a sensation that signals the urge for defecation. If environmental conditions are not conducive to defecation, voluntary contractions of the external sphincter can overcome the reflex. Relaxation of the internal sphincter is transient because the receptors within the rectal wall accommodate the stimulus of distention. Thus the internal anal sphincter regains its tone,

and the sensation subsides until the passage of more contents into the rectum. The rectum can accommodate rather large quantities of material, so it acts as a storage organ.

If the rectosphincteric reflex is elicited at a time when evacuation is convenient, defecation will occur. **Defecation** is accomplished by a series of voluntary and involuntary acts. When rectal distention is followed by defecation, muscles of the descending and sigmoid colon and the rectum may contract to propel contents toward the anal canal. Then both internal and external sphincters relax to allow passage of the bolus.

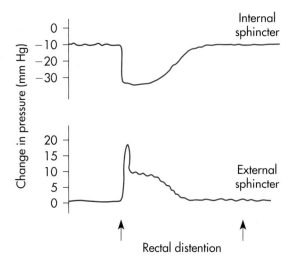

Figure 6-4 ■ Intraluminal pressure recorded at the level of the internal and external anal sphincters. Rectal distention causes relaxation of the internal sphincter and contraction of the external sphincter. Note, however, that the changes in sphincteric pressures are transient even though rectal distention is maintained. This is related to the accommodation of the stretch receptors within the wall of the rectum. (Modified from Schuster MM et al: Simultaneous manometric recording of internal and external anal sphincteric reflexes, *Johns Hopkins Med J* 116:70-88, 1965.)

Normally these events are accompanied by voluntary acts that raise intraabdominal pressure and lower the pelvic floor. Intraabdominal pressure is increased by contractions of the diaphragm and musculature of the abdominal wall. Simultaneously the musculature of the pelvic floor relaxes to allow the increased abdominal pressure to force the floor downward.

■ CONTROL OF MOTILITY

Factors that control motility of the large intestine are complex and poorly understood. As in the stomach and small intestine, motility in the large intestine is influenced by at least four factors: interstitial cells of Cajal–smooth muscle properties, enteric nerves, extrinsic nerves, and circulating or locally released chemicals.

Tone of the ileocecal sphincter is basically myogenic. It is modified, however, by nervous and humoral factors. Distention of the colon causes an increase in sphincteric tension, a reflex probably mediated via the enteric nerves (Figure 6-2, *B*). Distention of the ileum causes relaxation, also probably mediated via the enteric nerves (Figure 6-2, *A*). Relaxation of the sphincter and an increase in the contractile activity of the ileum occur with or shortly after eating. This has been termed the **gastroileal reflex.** One view is that the reflex is mediated by the gastrointestinal (GI) hormones, primarily gastrin and cholecystokinin (CCK). Both of these hormones will cause an increase in the contractile activity of the ileum, as well as a relaxation of the ileocecal sphincter. Some investigators, however, think that this reflex is mediated via the extrinsic autonomic nerves to the intestine.

Smooth muscle cells of the ascending, transverse, descending, and sigmoid colon and of the rectum exhibit fluctuations in their membrane potential. Cyclic depolarizations and repolarizations that possess some of the characteristics of small intestinal slow waves can be recorded. As in the small intestine, these slow waves are thought to depend upon interactions between smooth muscle cells and interstitial cells of Cajal. Potential changes that resemble spike potentials also are recorded. These probably initiate contractions, but the exact relationships between changes in potential and contractile activity have not been clarified. In addition, investigators have recorded various oscillations in membrane potential that fit descriptions of neither slow wave nor spike potential activities. Their origin and function are less clear.

Enteric neurons probably are involved in the control of colonic contractions. A peristaltic reflex can be initiated in the colon, and this reflex is mediated by nerve elements within the myenteric plexus. These plexal nerves seem to be predominantly inhibitory because in their absence the colon is contracted tonically. A number of colonic reflexes have their pathways in the extrinsic nerves. Distention of remote areas of the bowel induces an inhibition of contractions. The pathway for this reflex includes the inferior mesenteric ganglion and also may include the spinal cord. In addition, several investigations have demonstrated that the emotional state of an individual has a marked influence on colonic motility. These influences of the central nervous system are mediated by the extrinsic nerves.

The GI hormones, as well as epinephrine and the prostaglandins, affect colonic motility. Gastrin and CCK cause increases in colonic activity and have been implicated in the mass movement that sometimes is seen after eating. Epinephrine causes inhibition of all contractile activity, whereas the prostaglandins (primarily E type) cause a decrease in segmenting contractions and an increase in propulsive activity. The importance of these agents in regulating colonic motility is not known.

The rectosphincteric reflex and the act of defecation are under neural control. Part of the control lies in the enteric nervous system. The reflex, however, is reinforced by activity of neurons within the spinal cord. Destruction of the nerves to the anorectal area can result in fecal retention. The sensation of rectal distention, as well as voluntary control of the external anal sphincter, is mediated by pathways within the spinal cord to the cerebral cortex. Destruction of these pathways will lead to a loss of voluntary control of defecation.

■ CLINICAL SIGNIFICANCE

Abnormal transit of material through the colon is common. Delayed transit leads to **constipation;** in most situations, however, this is dietary in origin. There is a direct correlation between increased dietary fiber, increased colonic intraluminal bulk, and enhanced transit through the colon. How motility of the colon contributes to these changes in transit is not known. A particularly interesting and dramatic clinical disorder in which severe constipation is seen is congenital megacolon **(Hirschsprung's disease),** characterized by an absence of the enteric nervous system in the distal colon. The internal anal sphincter always is involved, and often the disease extends proximally into the rectum. The involved segment exhibits increased tone, has a very narrow lumen, and is devoid of propulsive activity. As a result, the colon proximal to the diseased segment becomes dilated, thus producing a megacolon. This condition is treated through surgical removal of the diseased segment.

In adults, the most common GI disorder for which medical advice is sought is the **irritable bowel syndrome.** This disorder gives rise most often to abdominal pain and altered bowel habit (constipation and/or diarrhea). In limited observations, exaggerated segmental contractions in the sigmoid colon have been seen, particularly in response to stimulants such as morphine. During stress, patients with irritable bowel syndrome and constipation exhibit increased segmentation in the sigmoid colon, whereas those with diarrhea exhibit decreased segmentation. The cause of this disorder remains unknown. One theory suggests that altered motility may reflect the conditioning of autonomic responses from repeated exposure to stressful situations. Other investigators have suggested changes in myoelectric activity that might render the colon more susceptible to exogenous influences (stress, drugs, hormones, etc.).

In older age groups, **diverticula** (outpouchings of mucosa that extend through the muscular wall) frequently develop in the colon. There is evidence to suggest that abnormal colonic motility leads to diverticula formation because of the generation of increased intraluminal pressure. However, a direct correlation between abnormal motility, symptoms, and the presence of diverticula cannot always be demonstrated.

■ **CLINICAL TESTS**

Despite the large numbers of patients in whom disordered colonic motility is suspected, techniques for monitoring contractions are not in general clinical use. Most often, radiologic procedures are used to provide limited information. In one test, radiopaque markers are ingested daily for 3 days. On the fourth day, a radiograph is taken and the number of markers in each region of the colon is noted and compared with normal values. Measurements of intraluminal pressures and myoelectric activity are feasible, especially in the sigmoid colon and rectum, because these areas are readily accessible. To date, such techniques are being used only in investigative studies; their usefulness in diagnosis and the assessment of treatment has yet to be proved.

The behavior of both the internal and the external anal sphincter, and the response to rectal distention, can be measured by the careful placement of small intraluminal balloons in the anal canal. A third balloon is placed in the rectum and distended to monitor the components of the defecation reflex. This technique has usefulness in patients with suspected neurologic disorders that result in impaired defecation.

■ **SUMMARY**

1. The muscular anatomy of the colon is characterized by concentration of the longitudinal muscle into bands called taeniae coli. Contraction of the taeniae coli and of the circular muscle results in haustrations.

2. The majority of colonic contractions are of the segmenting type that aid in the absorption of water and electrolytes. The frequency of segmenting contractions is higher in the descending and sigmoid colon than in more orad areas. This retards aboral progression.

3. Aboral movement of contents is slow, usually taking days to pass through the colon. Most aboral movement takes place during infrequent peristaltic contractions called mass movements.

4. Tonic contraction of the internal anal sphincter maintains closure of the anal canal. Distention of the rectum elicits relaxation of the internal anal sphincter and the sensation of the urge to defecate. Defecation can be prevented by voluntary contraction of the external anal sphincter while the rectum accommodates to the distention and the internal anal sphincter regains its tone. Relaxation of the external anal sphincter during this time leads to defecation.

5. Colonic slow waves are cyclic depolarizations and repolarizations of muscle cell membranes that appear to set the timing of segmental contractions. Neural activity and hormone levels influence the intensity of segmental contractions.

6. Mass movements are regulated by activities of the intrinsic and extrinsic nerves and possibly by the hormones gastrin and CCK. The rectosphincteric reflex is regulated by intrinsic nerves and by both extrinsic autonomic and somatic nerves.

■ **KEY WORDS AND CONCEPTS**

- Cecum
- Ascending, transverse, descending, and sigmoid colon
- Rectum
- Anal canal
- Taeniae coli
- External anal sphincter
- Haustra or haustrations
- Shunt fascicles
- Ileocecal junction
- Mass movement

- Rectosphincteric reflex
- Defecation
- Gastroileal reflex
- Constipation
- Hirschsprung's disease
- Irritable bowel syndrome
- Diverticula

■ BIBLIOGRAPHY

Christensen J: The motility of the colon. In Johnson LR, editor: *Physiology of the gastrointestinal tract,* vol 1, ed 3, New York, 1994, Raven Press.

Phillips SF: Motility disorders of the colon. In Yamada T, editor: *Textbook of gastroenterology,* vol 2, ed 2, Philadelphia, 1995, JB Lippincott.

Smith TK, Sanders KM: Motility of the large intestine. In Yamada T, editor: *Textbook of gastroenterology,* vol 1, ed 2, Philadelphia, 1995, JB Lippincott.

Salivary Secretion

Leonard R. Johnson

Although the salivary glands are not essential to life, their secretions are important to the hygiene and comfort of the mouth and teeth. The functions of saliva may be divided into those concerned with **lubrication, protection,** and **digestion.** An active process produces saliva in large quantities relative to the weights of the salivary glands. Saliva is hyposmotic at all rates of secretion, and unlike the other gastrointestinal (GI) secretions, the rate of secretion is almost totally under the control of the nervous system. Another characteristic of this regulation is that both branches of the autonomic nervous system (ANS) stimulate secretion. The parasympathetic system, however, provides a much greater stimulus than does the sympathetic.

■ FUNCTIONS OF SALIVA

The lubricating ability of saliva depends primarily on its content of **mucus.** In the mouth, mixing saliva with food lubricates the ingested material and facilitates the swallowing process. The lubricating effect of saliva is also necessary for speech, as evidenced by the glass of water normally found on the podium of a public speaker.

Saliva exerts its effects through a variety of different mechanisms. It protects the mouth by buffering and diluting noxious substances. Hot solutions of tea, coffee, or soup, for example, are diluted and cooled by saliva. Foul-tasting substances can be washed from the mouth by copious salivation. Similarly, the salivary glands are stimulated strongly before vomiting. The corrosive gastric acid and pepsin that are brought up into the esophagus and mouth are thereby neutralized and diluted by saliva. Dry mouth, or xerostomia, is associated with chronic infections of the buccal mucosa and with dental caries. Saliva dissolves and washes out food particles from between the teeth. A number of specialized constituents of saliva have antibacterial actions. These include a **lysozyme** that attacks bacterial cell walls; **lactoferrin,** which chelates iron, preventing the multiplication of organisms that require it for growth; and the **binding glycoprotein for immunoglobulin A** (IgA), which with IgA forms secretory IgA that in turn is immunologically active against viruses and bacteria. Various inorganic compounds are taken up by the salivary glands, concentrated, and secreted in saliva. These include substances such as fluoride and calcium, which subsequently are incorporated into the teeth.

The contributions made by saliva to normal digestion include dissolving and washing away food particles on the taste buds to enable one to taste the next morsel of food eaten. Saliva contains two enzymes, one directed toward carbohydrates and the other toward fat. An **α-amylase,** called **ptyalin,** cleaves internal α-1,4-glycosidic bonds present in starch. Exhaustive digestion of starch by this enzyme, which is identical to pancreatic amylase, produces maltose, maltotriose, and α-limit dextrins, which contain the α-1,6 branch points of the original molecule. Salivary amylase has a pH optimum of 7, and it is rapidly denatured at pH 4. However, because a large portion of a meal often remains unmixed for a considerable length of time in the orad stomach, the salivary enzyme may account for the digestion of as much as 75% of the starch present before it is denatured by gastric acid. In the absence of salivary amylase there is no defect in carbohydrate digestion, for the pancreatic enzyme is secreted in amounts sufficient to digest all of the starch present.

The serous salivary glands of the tongue secrete the second digestive enzyme, **lingual lipase,** which plays a role in the hydrolysis of dietary lipid. Unlike pancreatic lipase its properties allow it to act in all parts of the upper GI tract. Thus the ability of lingual lipase to hydrolyze lipids is not affected by surface-active detergents such as bile salts, medium chain fatty acids, and lecithin. It has an acidic pH optimum and remains active through the stomach and into the intestine.

■ ANATOMY AND INNERVATION OF THE SALIVARY GLANDS

The salivary glands are a collection of somewhat dissimilar structures in the mouth that produce a common juice, the saliva, although the composition of the secretion from different salivary glands differs. The largest of the salivary structures are the paired **parotid glands,** located near the angle of the jaw and the ear. They secrete a fairly watery juice, whereas the smaller bilateral **submandibular and sublingual glands** elaborate a more viscid saliva. Other still smaller glands occur in the mucosa covering the palate, buccal areas, lips, and tongue.

Most of the salivary glands are ectodermal in origin. The combined secretion of the parotid and submandibular glands constitutes 90% of the volume of saliva, which in a normal adult amounts to a half liter daily. The specific gravity of this mixed juice ranges from 1.000 to 1.010.

The microscopic structure of the salivary glands combines many features observed in another exocrine gland, the pancreas. A salivary gland consists of a blind-end system of microscopic ducts that branch out from grossly visible ducts. One main duct opens into the mouth from each gland. The functional unit of the salivary duct system, the **salivon,** is depicted in Figure 7-1. At the blind end is the **acinus,** surrounded by polygonal acinar cells. These cells secrete the initial saliva, including water, electrolytes, and organic molecules such as amylase. Sodium and water follow the chloride. Subsequently, the solutes and fluid diffuse out of the acinar cell into the duct lumen to form the initial saliva. The acinar cells are surrounded, in turn, by **myoepithelial cells.** The myoepithelial cells rest upon the basement membrane of acinar cells. They contain an actinomycin and have motile extensions. The next segment of the salivon is the **intercalated duct,** which may be associated with additional myoepithelial cells. Contraction of myoepithelial cells serves to expel formed saliva from the acinus, oppose retrograde movement of the juice during active secretion of saliva, shorten and widen the internal diameter of the intercalated duct (thereby lowering resistance to the flowing saliva), and prevent distention of the acinus (distention of the blind end of the salivon would permit back-diffusion of formed saliva through the stretched surface of the acinus). Whenever there

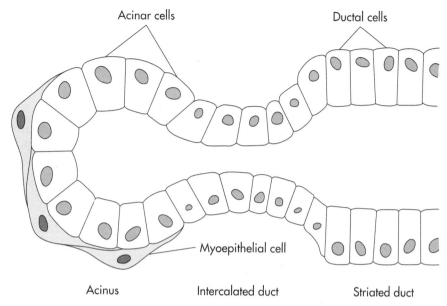

Acinar cells

Ductal cells

Myoepithelial cell

Acinus   Intercalated duct   Striated duct

Figure 7-1 ■ Cells lining the various portions of the salivon.

is an abrupt need for saliva in the mouth, as immediately before vomiting, myoepithelial contraction propels the secretion into the main duct of the gland. Other exocrine glands, such as the mammary glands and the pancreas, also possess myoepithelial cells.

The intercalated duct soon widens to become the **striated duct,** lined by columnar epithelial cells that resemble the epithelial components of the renal tubule in both shape and function. The saliva in the intercalated duct is similar in ionic composition to plasma. Changes from that composition occur because of ion exchanges in the striated duct. As saliva traverses the striated duct, sodium is actively resorbed from the juice, and potassium is transported into it. Calcium also enters secreting duct cells during salivation. Similarly, there is anionic exchange, with chloride being resorbed from the saliva and bicarbonate being added to it.

The striated duct epithelium is considered to be a fairly "tight" sheet membrane; that is, its surface is fairly impermeable to the back-diffusion of water from saliva into tissue, and osmotic gradients can be developed between saliva and interstitial fluid during secretion of potassium into the juice. These osmotic gradients draw water into the saliva from the tissue.

The blood supplied to the salivary glands is distributed by branches of the external carotid artery. The direction of arterial flow within the substance of each salivary gland is opposite the direction of flowing saliva within the ducts of each salivon. The arterioles break up into capillaries around acini and in nonacinar areas as well. Blood from nonacinar areas passes through portal venules back to the acinar capillaries, from which a second set of venules then drains all the blood to the systemic venous circulation. The rate of blood flow through resting salivary tissue is approximately 20 times that through muscle. This in part accounts for the prodigious amounts of saliva produced relative to the weights of the glands.

Both components of the ANS reach the salivary glands. The parasympathetic preganglionic fibers are delivered by the facial and glossopharyngeal nerves to autonomic ganglia, from which the postganglionic fibers pass to individual glands. The sympathetic preganglionic nerves originate at the cervical ganglion, whose postganglionic fibers extend to the gland in the periarterial spaces. These relationships appear in Figure 7-2. Parasympathetic and sympathetic mediators regulate all known salivary gland functions to an extraordinary degree. Their influence includes major effects upon not only secretion but also blood flow, ductular smooth muscle activity, growth, and metabolism of the salivary glands.

■ COMPOSITION OF SALIVA

The major constituents of saliva are water, electrolytes, and a few enzymes. The **unique properties** of this GI juice are: (1) its large volume relative to the mass of glands that secrete saliva; (2) its low osmolality; (3) its high potassium concentration; and (4) the specific organic materials it contains.

Inorganic Composition

Compared with other secretory organs of the GI tract, the salivary glands elaborate a remarkably large volume of juice per gram of tissue. Thus, for example, an entire pancreas may reach a maximal rate of secretion of 1 ml/min, whereas at highest rates of secretion in some animals, a tiny submaxillary gland can secrete 1 ml/g/min, a fiftyfold higher rate. In humans, the salivary glands secrete at rates severalfold higher than other GI organs per unit weight of tissue.

The osmolality of saliva is significantly lower than that of plasma at all but the highest rates of secretion, when the saliva becomes isotonic with plasma. As the secretory rate of the salivon increases, the osmolality of its saliva also increases.

The concentrations of electrolytes in saliva vary with the rate of secretion (Figure 7-3). The potassium concentration of saliva is 2 to 30 times

that of the plasma, depending on the rate of secretion, the nature of the stimulus, the plasma potassium concentration, and the level of mineralocorticoids in the circulation. Saliva has the highest potassium concentration of any digestive juice; maximal concentration values approach those within cells. These remarkable levels of salivary potassium imply the existence of an energy-dependent transport mechanism within the salivon. In most species the concentration of Na^+ in saliva is always less than that in plasma, and, as the secretory rate increases, the Na^+ concentration also increases. In general, Cl^- concentrations parallel those of Na^+. These findings suggest that Na^+ and Cl^- are secreted and then reabsorbed as the saliva passes through the ducts. The concentration of HCO_3^- in saliva is higher than that in plasma, except at low flow rates. This also accounts for the changes in the pH of saliva. At basal rates of flow the pH is slightly acidic but rapidly rises to around 8 as flow is stimulated. The relationships between ion concentrations and flow rates shown in Figure 7-3 will vary somewhat depending on the stimulus.

The relationships shown in Figure 7-3 are explained by two basic types of studies that indicate how the final saliva is produced. First, fluid collected by micropuncture of the intercalated ducts contains Na^+, K^+, Cl^-, and HCO_3^- in concentrations approximately equal to their plasma concentrations. This fluid is also isotonic to plasma. Second, if one perfuses a salivary gland duct with fluid containing ions in concentrations similar to those of plasma, Na^+ and Cl^- concentrations are decreased and the K^+ and HCO_3^- concentrations are increased when the fluid is collected at the duct opening. The fluid also becomes hypotonic, and the longer the fluid remains in the duct (i.e., the slower the rate of perfusion) the greater the changes. These data indicate, first, that the acini secrete a fluid similar to plasma in its concentration of ions, and, second, that as the fluid moves down the duct, Na^+ and Cl^- are reabsorbed and K^+ and HCO_3^- are se-

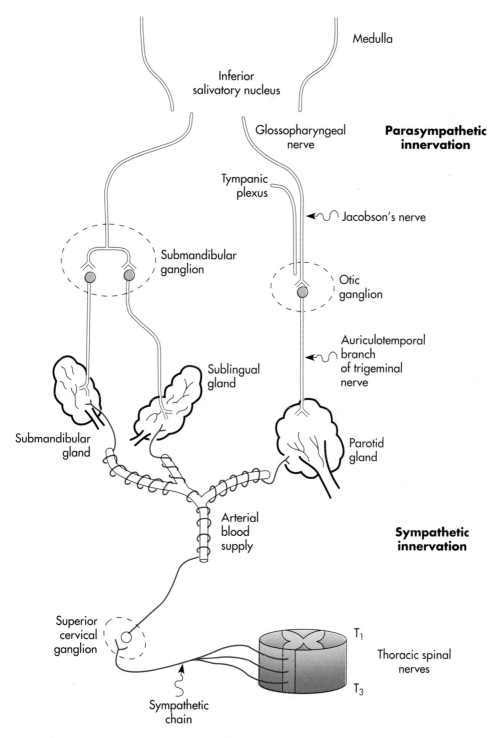

Figure 7-2 ■ Autonomic nervous distribution to the major salivary glands.

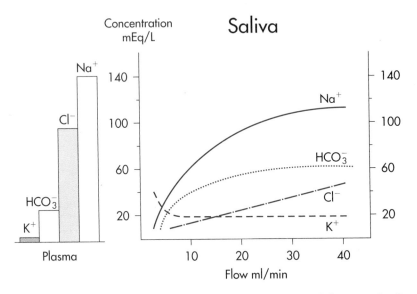

Figure 7-3 ■ Concentrations of major ions in the saliva as a function of the rate of salivary secretion. Values in plasma are shown for comparison.

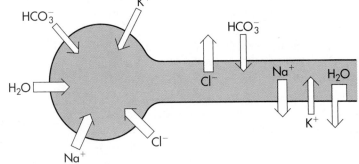

Figure 7-4 ■ Movements of ions and water in the acinus and duct of the salivon.

creted into the saliva. The higher the flow of saliva, the less time is available for modification, and the final saliva more closely resembles plasma in its ionic makeup (Figure 7-3). At low flow rates K^+ increases considerably and Na^+ and Cl^- decrease. Because most salivary agonists stimulate HCO_3^- secretion, the HCO_3^- concentration remains relatively high even at high rates of secretion. Some K^+ and HCO_3^- are reabsorbed in

exchange for Na^+ and Cl^-, but much more Na^+ and Cl^- leave the duct and the saliva becomes hypotonic. Because the duct epithelium is relatively impermeable to water, the final product remains hypotonic. These processes are depicted in Figure 7-4.

Current evidence indicates that Cl^- is the primary ion that is actively secreted by the acinar cells (Figure 7-5). No evidence exists for direct active secretion of Na$^+$. The secretory mechanism for Cl$^-$ is inhibited by ouabain, indicating that it depends on the Na$^+$-K$^+$ pump in the basolateral membrane. The active pumping of Na$^+$ out of the cell creates a diffusion gradient for Na$^+$ to enter across the basolateral membrane. Cl$^-$ is cotransported with Na$^+$ into the cell to preserve electrical neutrality. This increases the electrochemical potential of Cl$^-$ within the cell, and Cl$^-$ diffuses down this gradient into the lumen via an electrogenic ion channel that also allows HCO$_3^-$ to enter the lumen. The secretion of HCO$_3^-$ is facilitated by the movement of H$^+$ out of the cell in exchange for Na$^+$. Na$^+$ moves paracellularly, through the tight junctions, into the lumen preserving electroneutrality; and water follows down its osmotic gradient. There is now evidence for a Ca^{++}-activated K$^+$ channel in the basolateral membrane. Exodus of K$^+$ increases the electronegativity of the cytosol, increasing the driving force for the entry of Cl$^-$ and HCO$_3^-$ into the lumen. Agents that stimulate salivary secretion increase the activity of all these channels and transport processes.

Within the ducts (Figure 7-5), Na$^+$ is actively absorbed and K$^+$ is actively secreted. These processes depend on several transporters that are powered by the Na$^+$ gradient created by the Na$^+$, K$^+$-ATPase in the basolateral membrane. The apical membrane contains Na$^+$-H$^+$ and Cl$^-$-HCO$_3^-$ exchangers that result in the electroneutral uptake of NaCl. The Na$^+$ is pumped out of the cell by the ATPase, and Cl$^-$ exits the basolateral surface via an electrogenic Cl$^-$ channel. Some K$^+$ also enters the cell through a basolateral channel to balance the movement of Cl$^-$. K$^+$ enters the lumen in exchange for H$^+$. A Na$^+$-H$^+$ exchanger in the basolateral membrane increases the pH of the cell, driving the Cl$^-$-HCO$_3^-$ exchange at the apical membrane. The tight junctions of the ductule epithelium are relatively impermeable to water compared with those of the acini. The net result is a decrease in Na$^+$ and Cl$^-$ concentrations and an increase in K$^+$ and HCO$_3^-$ concentrations

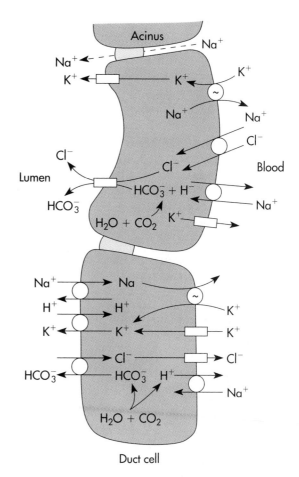

= passive conductance

= Secondary active transport

= Primary active transport

Figure 7-5 ■ **Intracellular mechanisms for the movement of ions in acinar and ductule cells of the salivary glands.**

and pH as the saliva moves down the duct. More ions leave than H$_2$O, and the saliva becomes hypotonic. Aldosterone acts at the luminal membrane to increase the absorption of Na$^+$ and the secretion of K$^+$.

Organic Composition

Some organic materials produced and secreted by the salivary glands have been mentioned already in the section describing the functions of saliva. These include the enzymes α-amylase (ptyalin) and lingual lipase, mucus, glycoproteins, lysozymes, and lactoferrin. Another enzyme produced by salivary glands is **kallikrein,** which converts a plasma protein into the potent vasodilator **bradykinin.** Kallikrein is released when the metabolism of the salivary glands increases; it is responsible in part for increased blood flow to the secreting glands. Saliva also contains the blood group substances, A, B, AB, O.

The synthesis of salivary gland enzymes, their storage, and their release are similar to the same processes in the pancreas, which are detailed in Chapter 9. The protein concentration of saliva is about one-tenth the concentration of proteins in the plasma.

■ REGULATION OF SALIVARY SECRETION

The ANS controls essentially all salivary gland secretion. Antidiuretic hormone (ADH, vasopressin) and aldosterone modify the composition of saliva by decreasing its Na^+ concentrations and increasing its K^+ concentrations, but they do not regulate the flow of saliva. The absence of hormonal control of salivation contrasts with the regulation of the flow of gastric and pancreatic juice and bile. The GI hormones exert major influences on the secretory activity of the stomach, pancreas, and liver. Control of the salivary glands is also unusual in that both the parasympathetic and sympathetic branches stimulate secretion. The parasympathetic system, however, exerts a much greater influence.

Stimulation of the parasympathetic nerves to the salivary glands begins and maintains salivary secretion. Increased secretion results from the activation of transport processes in both acinar and duct cells. Secretion is enhanced by the contraction of the myoepithelial cells that are innervated by the parasympathetic nerves. Parasympathetic fibers also innervate the surrounding blood vessels, stimulating vasodilation and increasing blood flow to the secreting cells. Increased cellular activity in response to parasympathetic stimulation results in increased consumption of glucose and oxygen and the production of vasodilator metabolites. In addition, kallikrein is released, resulting in the production of the potent vasodilator bradykinin. Increased cellular activity eventually results in growth of the salivary glands. Section of the parasympathetic nerves to the salivary glands causes the glands to atrophy. These processes are outlined in Figure 7-6.

Sympathetic activation also stimulates secretion, myoepithelial cell contraction, metabolism, and growth of the salivary glands, although these effects are less pronounced and of shorter duration than those produced by the parasympathetics. Stimulation via the sympathetic nerves produces a biphasic change in blood flow to the salivary glands. The earliest response is a decrease caused by activation of α-adrenergic receptors and vasoconstriction. However, as vasodilator metabolites are produced, blood flow increases over resting levels. Section of the sympathetic fibers to the salivary glands, unlike section of the parasympathetic fibers, has little effect. The effects of sympathetic stimulation also are summarized in Figure 7-6.

Salivary glands contain receptors to many mediators, but the most important functionally are the muscarinic cholinergic and β-adrenergic receptors. The parasympathetic mediator is acetylcholine, which acts on muscarinic receptors, resulting in the formation of inositol triphosphate (IP_3) and the subsequent release of Ca^{++} from intercellular stores. Ca^{++} also may enter the cell from outside. Other agents that are released from neurons in salivary glands and that release Ca^{++} include vasoactive intestinal peptide and substance P. The primary sympathetic mediator is

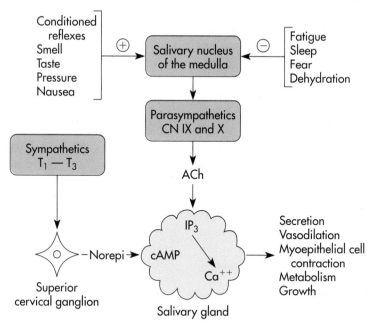

Figure 7-6 ■ Summary of the regulation of salivary gland function.

norepinephrine, which binds to β-adrenergic receptors resulting in the formation of cyclic adenosine monophosphate (cAMP). Formation of these second messengers results in protein phosphorylation and enzyme activation that ultimately leads to the stimulation of the salivary glands. In general, agonists that release Ca^{++} have a greater effect on the volume of acinar cell secretion, while those elevating cAMP lead to a greater increase in enzyme and mucus content.

The dual autonomic regulation of the salivary glands is unusual in that the parasympathetic and sympathetic systems both stimulate secretory, metabolic, trophic, muscular, and circulatory functions in similar directions. Their complementary effects are shown in Figure 7-6.

Ultimately, the central nervous system and its autonomic arms are what respond to external events and either stimulate or inhibit activities of the salivary glands. Common events leading to increased glandular activities include chewing,

consuming spicy or sour-tasting foods, and smoking. External events leading to glandular inhibition include sleep, fear, dehydration, and fatigue. Glandular activities sensitive to neural control include secretion, circulation, myoepithelial contraction, cellular metabolism, and even parenchymal growth.

Medical events likewise can alter either the amount or the composition of saliva. Besides congenital xerostomia (absence of saliva), there is Sjögren's syndrome, an acquired disease characterized by atrophy of the glands and decreased salivation. The commonly used drugs of the digitalis family cause increased concentrations of calcium and potassium in saliva. In cystic fibrosis, salivary sodium, calcium, and protein are elevated (as are these components in the bronchial secretions, pancreatic juice, and sweat of these patients). Salivary sodium concentrations also are elevated in Addison's disease, though they are decreased in Cushing's syndrome, in primary aldosteronism, and during pregnancy. These elec-trolytic changes in saliva reflect events or dis-eases that make similar alterations in other bodily secretions. Excessive salivation is observed with tumors of the mouth or esophagus and with Parkinson's disease. In these cases, unusual local, reflexive, and more general neurologic stimuli are responsible.

■ SUMMARY

1. The functions of saliva include those con-cerned with digestion, protection, and lubri-cation.
2. Saliva is noteworthy in that it is produced in large volumes relative to the weight of the glands, is hypotonic, and contains relatively high concentrations of K^+.
3. The primary saliva is produced in end pieces called acini and is then modified as it passes through the ducts.
4. Acinar secretion contains ions and water in concentrations approximately equal to those in plasma.
5. Within the ducts Na^+ and Cl^- are reabsorbed, and K^+ and HCO_3^- are secreted.
6. Since the ductule epithelium is relatively im-permeable to water and ions, the saliva be-comes more hypotonic as it moves through the ducts.
7. All regulatory control of salivation is provided by the ANS, and both the parasympathetic and sympathetic branches stimulate secretion and metabolism of the glands.

■ KEY WORDS AND CONCEPTS

- Lubricative function of saliva
- Protective function of saliva
- Digestive function of saliva
- Mucus
- Lysozyme
- Lactoferrin
- Binding glycoprotein for immunoglobulin A
- α-amylase
- Ptyalin
- Lingual lipase
- Parotid glands
- Submandibular and sublingual glands
- Salivon
- Acinus
- Myoepithelial cells
- Intercalated duct
- Striated duct
- Unique properties of saliva
- Kallikrein
- Bradykinin

■ BIBLIOGRAPHY

Cook DI, van Lennep EW, Roberts M, Young JA: Secretion by the major salivary glands. In Johnson LR, editor: *Physiology of the gastrointestinal tract,* ed 3, New York, 1994, Raven Press.

Gastric Secretion

Leonard R. Johnson

our constituents of gastric juice—**intrinsic factor, hydrogen ion, pepsin,** and **mucus**—have physiologic functions. They are secreted by the various cells present within the gastric mucosa. The only indispensable ingredient in gastric juice is intrinsic factor, required for the absorption of vitamin B_{12} by the ileal mucosa. Acid is necessary for the conversion of inactive pepsinogen to the enzyme pepsin. Acid and pepsin begin the digestion of protein, but in their absence pancreatic enzymes hydrolyze all ingested protein, so no nitrogen is wasted in the stools. Acid also kills a large number of bacteria that enter the stomach, thereby reducing the number of organisms reaching the intestine. In cases of severely reduced or absent acid secretion, the incidence of intestinal infections is greater. Mucus lines the wall of the stomach, protecting it from damage. It acts primarily as a lubricant, protecting the mucosa from physical injury. Together with HCO_3^-, mucus neutralizes acid and maintains the surface of the mucosa at a pH near neutrality. This is part of the **gastric mucosal barrier** that protects the stomach from acid and pepsin digestion.

Gastric juice and many of its functions originally were described by a young army surgeon,

William Beaumont, stationed at a fort on Mackinac Island in northern Michigan. Beaumont was called to treat a French Canadian, Alexis St. Martin, who had been shot accidentally in the side at close range with a shotgun. St. Martin unexpectedly survived but was left with a permanent opening into his stomach from the outside (gastric fistula). The accident occurred in 1822, and during the ensuing 3 years Beaumont nursed St. Martin back to health. Beaumont retained St. Martin "for the purpose of making physiological experiments," which were begun in 1825. Beaumont's observations and conclusions, many of which remain unchanged today, included a description of the juice itself and its digestive and bacteriostatic functions, the identification of the acid as hydrochloric, the realization that mucus was a separate secretion, the realization that mental disturbances affected gastric function, a direct study of gastric motility, and a thorough study of the ability of gastric juices to digest various foodstuffs.

■ FUNCTIONAL ANATOMY

Functionally, the gastric mucosa is divided into the **oxyntic gland area** and the **pyloric gland area** (Figure 8-1). The oxyntic gland mucosa se-

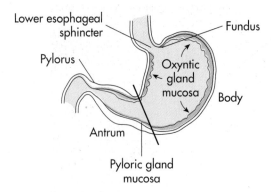

Figure 8-1 ■ **Areas of the stomach.**

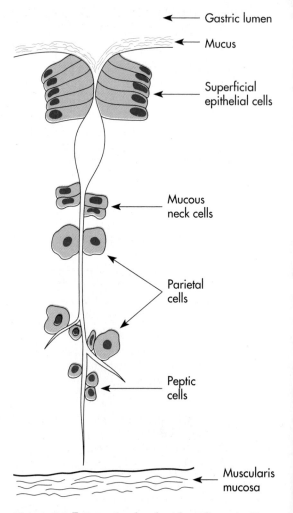

Figure 8-2 ■ **Oxyntic gland and surface pit. Note the positions of the various cell types.**

cretes acid and is located in the proximal 80% of the stomach. It includes the body and the fundus. The distal 20% of the gastric mucosa, referred to as the pyloric gland mucosa, synthesizes and releases the hormone gastrin. This area of the stomach often is designated as the **antrum**.

The gastric mucosa is composed of pits and glands (Figure 8-2). The pits and surface itself are lined with mucous or surface epithelial cells. At the base of the pits are the openings of the glands, which project into the mucosa toward the outside or serosa. The oxyntic glands contain the acid-producing **parietal cells** and the **peptic or chief cells**, which secrete the enzyme precursor pepsinogen. Pyloric glands contain the gastrin-producing G cells and mucous cells, which also produce **pepsinogen**. Mucous neck cells are present where the glands open into the pits. Each gland contains a stem cell(s) (there may be only one per gland) in this region. These cells divide, and the daughter cells migrate both to the surface, where they differentiate into mucous cells, and down into the glands, where they become parietal cells in the oxyntic gland area. Endocrine cells such as the G cells also differentiate from stem cells. Peptic cells are capable of mitosis, but there is evidence that they also can arise from stem cells during the repair of damage to the mucosa. Cells of the surface and pits are replaced much more rapidly than are those of the glands.

The parietal cells secrete hydrochloric acid and, in humans, intrinsic factor. In some species the chief cells secrete intrinsic factor. The normal human stomach contains approximately 1 billion parietal cells, which produce acid at a concentration of 150 to 160 mEq/L. The number of parietal cells determines the maximal secretory rate and accounts for variability between in-

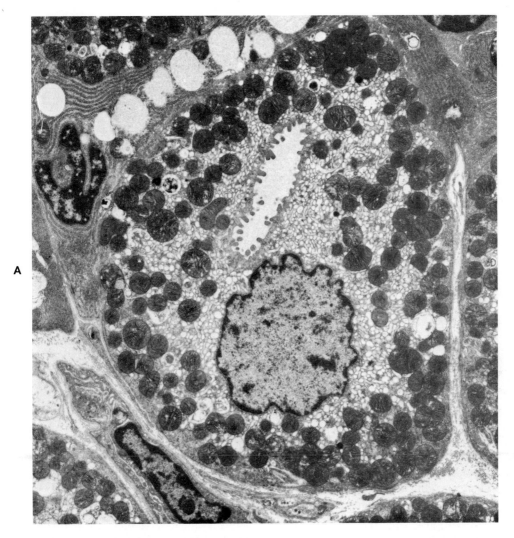

Figure 8-3 ■ Parietal cell. A, Electron photomicrograph. (A, Courtesy Dr. Bruce MacKay.)

Continued

dividuals. The human stomach secretes 1 to 2 L of gastric juice per day. Because the pH of the final juice at high rates of secretion may be less than 1 and that of the blood is 7.4, the parietal cells must expend a large amount of energy to concentrate hydrogen ions. The energy for the production of this more than a millionfold concentration gradient comes from adenosine triphosphate produced by the numerous mitochondria located within the cell (Figure 8-3).

During the resting state, the cytoplasm of the parietal cells is dominated by numerous **tubulovesicles**. There is also an **intracellular canaliculus** that is continuous with the lumen of the oxyntic gland. After stimulation of acid secretion, the tubulovesicles become microvilli and project

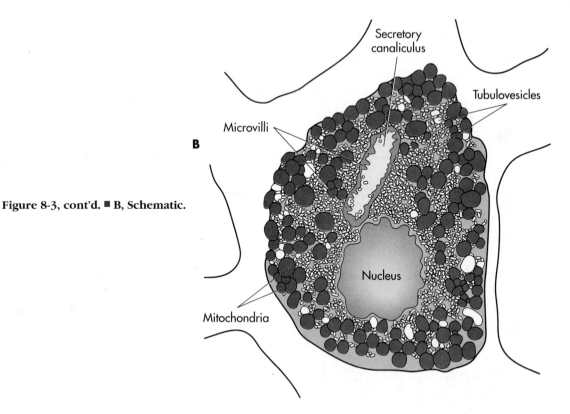

Figure 8-3, cont'd. ▪ B, Schematic.

into the canaliculus, which has become greatly expanded to occupy much of the cell. **Carbonic anhydrase** and **H⁺, K⁺-ATPase**, enzymes necessary for the production and secretion of acid, are localized in the microvilli. The activities of these enzymes increase during acid secretion. Acid secretion begins within 10 minutes of administering a stimulant. This lag time probably is expended in the morphological conversion and enzyme activations described previously.

The surface epithelial mucous cells are recognized primarily by the large number of mucous granules at their apical surfaces. During secretion, the membranes of the granules fuse with the cell membrane, expelling mucus.

Peptic cells contain a highly developed endoplasmic reticulum for the synthesis of pepsinogen. The proenzyme is packaged into zymogen granules by the numerous Golgi structures within the cytoplasm. The zymogen granules migrate to the apical surface, where, during secretion, they empty their contents into the lumen by exocytosis. This entire procedure of enzyme synthesis, packaging, and secretion is discussed in greater detail in Chapter 9.

Endocrine cells of the gut also contain numerous granules. However, unlike the peptic and mucous cells, these hormone-containing granules are located at the base of the cell. The hormones are secreted into the intercellular space, from which they diffuse into the capillaries. The endocrine cells have numerous microvilli extending from their apical surface into the lumen. Presumably the microvilli contain receptors that sample the luminal contents and trigger hormone secretion in response to the appropriate stimuli.

■ SECRETION OF ACID

The transport processes involved in the secretion of hydrochloric acid are shown in Figure 8-4. The exact biochemical steps for the production of H^+ are not known, but the reaction can be summarized as:

$$HOH \rightarrow OH^- + H^+ \qquad (1)$$

$$OH^- + CO_2 \overset{CA}{\rightarrow} HCO_3^- \qquad (2)$$

H^+ is pumped actively into the lumen and HCO_3^- diffuses into the blood, giving gastric venous blood a higher pH than arterial blood when the stomach is secreting. Step 2 is catalyzed by carbonic anhydrase. Inhibition of this enzyme decreases the rate but does not prevent acid secretion. Metabolism produces much of the CO_2 used to neutralize OH^-, but at high secretory rates CO_2 from the blood also is required. The active transport of H^+ across the mucosal membrane is catalyzed by H^+, K^+-ATPase, and H^+ is pumped into the lumen in exchange for K^+. Within the cell, K^+ is accumulated by the Na^+, K^+-ATPase in the basolateral membrane. Accumulated K^+ moves down its electrochemical gradient, leaking across both membranes. Luminal K^+ is therefore recycled by the H^+, K^+-ATPase. Cl^- enters the cell across the basolateral membrane in exchange for HCO_3^-. The pumping of H^+ out of the cell allows OH^- to accumulate and form HCO_3^- from CO_2, a step catalyzed by carbonic anhydrase. The HCO_3^- entering the blood causes its pH to increase, so the gastric venous blood from the actively secreting stomach has a higher pH than arterial blood. The production of OH^- is facilitated by the low intracellular Na^+ concentration established by the Na^+, K^+-ATPase. Some Na^+ moves down its gradient back into the cell in exchange for H^+, further increasing OH^- production. This in turn increases HCO_3^- production, enhancing the driving force for the entry of Cl^- and its uphill movement from the blood into the lumen. Thus the movement of Cl^- from blood to lumen against both electrical and chemical gradients is the result of excess OH^- in the cell after the H^+ has been pumped out.

The H^+, K^+-ATPase catalyzes the pumping of H^+ out of the cytoplasm into the secretory canaliculus in exchange for K^+. In the resting cell, the H^+, K^+-ATPase is found in the membranes of the tubulovesicles. Following a secretory stimulus, the tubulovesicles fuse with the canaliculus, greatly increasing the surface area of the secretory membrane and the number of "pumps" in it. When acid secretion ends, the tubulovesicles reform and the canaliculus shrinks. There is some controversy over whether the tubulovesicles are separate structures or whether they are collapsed canalicular membrane. Most evidence, however, suggests they are separate structures that fuse with the canaliculus and undergo recycling following secretion. H^+, K^+-ATPase, like Na^+, K^+-ATPase, with which it has a 60% amino acid homology, is a member of the P-type ion transporting ATPases, which also include the Ca^{++}-ATPase. Inhibition of the H^+, K^+-

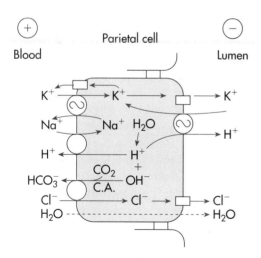

Figure 8-4 ■ Transport processes in the gastric mucosa accounting for the presence of the various ions in gastric juice and for the negative transmembrane potential.

ATPase totally blocks gastric acid secretion. Drugs such as omeprazole, a substituted benzimidazole, are accumulated in acid spaces and are activated at low pH. They then bind irreversibly to sulfhydryl groups of the H^+, K^+-ATPase, inactivating it. Omeprazole is the most potent of the different types of acid secretory inhibitors and is an effective agent in the treatment of peptic ulcer, even that caused by a gastrinoma (Zollinger-Ellison syndrome).

ORIGIN OF THE ELECTRICAL POTENTIAL DIFFERENCE

The potential difference across the resting oxyntic gland mucosa is -70 to -80 mV lumen negative with respect to the blood. This charge separation primarily is caused by the secretion of Cl^- (see previous section) against its electrochemical gradient. This is accomplished by both surface epithelial cells and parietal cells. Following the stimulation of acid secretion, the potential difference decreases to -30 or -40 mV because the positively charged H^+ moves in the same direction as Cl^-. H^+, therefore, actually is secreted down its electrical gradient, facilitating its transport against a several millionfold concentration gradient.

To produce an electrical gradient and a millionfold concentration gradient of H^+, there must be minimal leakage of ions and acid back into the mucosa. The ability of the stomach to prevent leakage is attributed to the so-called gastric mucosal barrier. If this barrier is disrupted by aspirin, alcohol, bile, or a number of agents that damage the gastric mucosa, the potential difference decreases as ions leak down their electrochemical gradients. The exact nature of the barrier is unknown; its properties and the consequences of disrupting it are discussed more fully in the section on the pathophysiology of ulcer diseases (p. 85). The negative potential difference across the stomach facilitates acid secretion because H^+ is secreted down the electrical gradient. The potential difference can be used to position catheters within the digestive tract. With an electrode placed at the catheter tip, the oxyntic gland mucosa can be distinguished readily from the esophagus (potential difference, -15 mV) or the duodenum (potential difference, -5 mV).

ELECTROLYTES OF GASTRIC JUICE

The concentrations of the major electrolytes in gastric juice are variable but usually are related to the rate of secretion (Figure 8-5). At low rates the final juice is essentially a solution of NaCl with small amounts of H^+ and K^+. As the rate increases, the concentration of Na^+ decreases and that of H^+ increases. The concentrations of both Cl^- and K^+ rise slightly as the secretory rate rises. At peak rates, gastric juice is primarily HCl with small amounts of Na^+ and K^+. At all rates of secretion, the concentrations of H^+, K^+, and Cl^- are higher than those in plasma, and the concentration of Na^+ is lower than that in plasma. Thus gastric juice and plasma—regardless of the secretory rate—are approximately isotonic.

To help understand the changes in ionic concentration, it is convenient to think of gastric juice as a mixture of two separate secretions: a nonparietal and a parietal component. The nonparietal component is a basal alkaline secretion of constant and low volume. Its primary constituents are Na^+ and Cl^-, and it contains K^+ at about the same concentration as does plasma. In the absence of H^+ secretion, HCO_3^- can be detected in gastric juice. The HCO_3^- is secreted at a concentration of about 30 mEq/L. The nonparietal component is always present, and the parietal component is secreted against this background. As the rate of secretion increases, and because the increase is caused solely by the parietal component, the concentrations of electrolytes in the final juice begin to approach those of pure parietal cell secretion. Pure parietal cell secretion is slightly hyperosmotic and contains

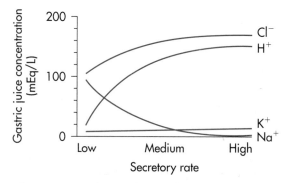

Figure 8-5 ■ Relationship of the electrolyte concentrations in gastric juice to the rate of gastric secretion.

150 to 160 mEq H^+/L and 10 to 20 mEq K^+/L. The only anion present is Cl^-.

This so-called two-component model of gastric secretion is an oversimplification. Parietal secretion is modified somewhat by the exchange of Na^+ for H^+ as the juice moves up the gland into the lumen. Although such changes are minimal, they do participate in determining the final ionic composition of gastric juice.

A knowledge of the composition of gastric juice is required to treat a patient with chronic vomiting or one whose gastric juice is being aspirated and who is being maintained intravenously. Replacement of only NaCl and dextrose will result in hypokalemic metabolic alkalosis, which can be fatal.

■ STIMULANTS OF ACID SECRETION

Only a few agents directly stimulate the parietal cells to secrete acid. The antral hormone gastrin and the parasympathetic mediator acetylcholine (ACh) are the most important physiologic regulators. ACh stimulates gastrin release in addition to stimulating the parietal cell directly.

Evidence has accumulated that an unknown hormone of intestinal origin also stimulates acid secretion. This substance tentatively has been named *enterooxyntin* to denote both its origin and its action. In humans, circulating amino acids also stimulate the parietal cell and provide some of the stimulation of acid secretion that results from the presence of food in the small intestine.

Histamine, which occurs in many tissues (including the entire gastrointestinal [GI] tract), is a potent stimulator of parietal cell secretion. There is evidence that histamine release is regulated by gastrin in most mammals and that it in turn stimulates acid secretion in the sense that gastrin and ACh do.

■ ROLE OF HISTAMINE IN ACID SECRETION

In 1920 a Polish physiologist, Popielski, discovered that histamine stimulated gastric acid secretion. It was then believed by many that gastrin was actually histamine. The confusion cleared somewhat in 1938 when Komarov demonstrated that there were two separate secretagogues in the gastric mucosa. He showed that trichloroacetic acid precipitated the peptide gastrin from gastric mucosal extracts, leaving histamine in the supernatant. It was then suggested by MacIntosh that histamine was the final common mediator of acid secretion. He proposed that gastrin and ACh released histamine, which in turn stimulated the parietal cells directly and was the only direct stimulant of the parietal cells.

At this point it is important to introduce and define the concept of **potentiation**. Potentiation is said to occur between two stimulants if the response to their simultaneous administration exceeds the sum of the responses when each is administered alone. A number of secretory responses in the GI tract depend on the potentiation of two or more agonists. In the stomach histamine potentiates the effects of gastrin and ACh on the parietal cell. ACh also potentiates the response to gastrin. In this way small amounts of stimuli acting together often can produce a near-maximal secretory response. Potentiation requires the presence of separate receptors on the target cell for each stimulant and, in the case of acid secretion, is incompatible with the final common mediator hypothesis.

Until recently all antihistamines blocked only the histamine H_1-receptor, which mediates actions such as bronchoconstriction and vasodilation. The stimulation of acid secretion by histamine is mediated by the H_2-receptor and is not blocked by conventional antihistamines. A new H_2-receptor antagonist, **cimetidine**, effectively inhibits histamine-stimulated acid secretion. Cimetidine, however, has been found also to inhibit the secretory responses to gastrin, ACh, and food. Atropine, a specific antagonist of the muscarinic actions of ACh, decreases the acid responses to gastrin and histamine as well as to ACh. When preparations of isolated parietal cells (which rule out the presence of stimuli other than those directly added) are used, it has been shown that some effects of cimetidine on gastrin- and ACh-stimulated secretion are caused by the inhibition of the part of the secretory response resulting from histamine potentiation. Similarly the inhibition of gastrin- and histamine-stimulated secretion by atropine is caused by removal of the potentiating effects of ACh. Cimetidine is a more effective inhibitor of acid secretion than atropine and has fewer side effects. It is an extremely effective drug for the treatment of duodenal ulcer disease.

Histamine is found in **enterochromaffin-like** (ECL) **cells** within the lamina propria of the gastric glands. The relationships between gastrin, histamine, and ACh are shown in Figure 8-6. Located close to the parietal cells, ECL cells release histamine that acts as a paracrine to stimulate acid secretion. ECL cells have receptors for gastrin and ACh. Gastrin stimulates histamine release and synthesis and the growth of the ECL cells. ACh also appears to stimulate histamine release. The parietal cell membrane contains receptors for all three agonists. Gastrin and ACh activate phospholipase C (PLC), which catalyzes

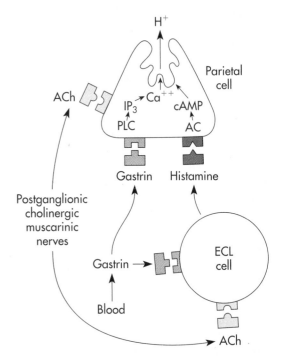

Figure 8-6 ■ The parietal cell contains receptors for gastrin, ACh, and histamine. In addition, gastrin and ACh release histamine from the ECL cell.

the formation of inositol triphosphate (IP_3). IP_3 causes the release of intracellular Ca^{++}. Histamine activates adenylate cyclase (AC) to form cyclic adenosine monophosphate (cAMP). Ca^{++} and cAMP trigger the events leading to secretion and potentiate each other's effects. Thus the inhibition of acid secretion by histamine H_2-antagonists, such as cimetidine, is due both to removal of potentiative interactions with histamine and inhibition of the stimulation caused by histamine released by gastrin.

■ STIMULATION OF ACID SECRETION

The unstimulated human stomach secretes acid at a rate equal to 10% to 15% of that present during maximal stimulation. Basal acid secretion exhibits a diurnal rhythm with higher rates in the evening and lower rates in the morning before awakening. The cause of the diurnal variation is unknown, since plasma gastrin is relatively constant during the interdigestive phase. The stomach emptied of food therefore contains a relatively small volume of gastric juice. The pH of this fluid is usually less than 2. Thus in the absence of food the gastric mucosa is acidified.

The stimulation of gastric secretion is conveniently divided into three phases based on the location of the receptors initiating the secretory responses. It is important to realize that this division is artificial; shortly after the start of a meal, stimulation is initiated from all three areas at the same time.

Cephalic Phase

Chemoreceptors and mechanoreceptors located in the tongue and the buccal and nasal cavities are stimulated by tasting, smelling, chewing, and swallowing food. The afferent nerve impulses are relayed through the vagal nucleus and vagal efferent fibers to the stomach. Even the thought of an appetizing meal stimulates gastric secretion. The secretory response to cephalic stimulation depends greatly on the nature of the meal. The greatest response occurs to an appetizing self-selected meal. A bland meal produces a much smaller response. The efferent pathway for the cephalic phase is the vagus nerve. The entire response is blocked by vagotomy.

The cephalic phase is best studied by the procedure known as sham-feeding. A dog is prepared with esophageal and gastric fistulas. When the esophageal fistula is open, swallowed food falls to the exterior without entering the stomach. Gastric secretion is collected from the gastric fistula, and its volume and acid content are measured. Stimulation during the cephalic phase represents about 30% of the total response to a meal. The cephalic phase also can be studied using a variety of drugs. Hypoglycemia introduced by tolbutamide or insulin, or interference with

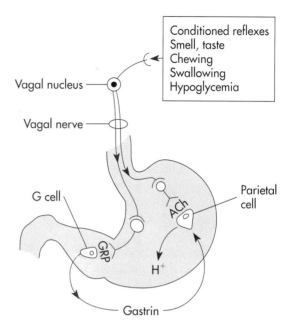

Figure 8-7 ■ Mechanisms stimulating gastric acid secretion during the cephalic phase.

glucose metabolism by glucose analogues such as 3-methylglucose or 2-deoxyglucose, activates hypothalamic centers that stimulate secretion via the vagus nerve.

The vagus acts directly on the parietal cells to stimulate acid secretion. It also acts upon the antral gastrin cells to stimulate gastrin release. The mediator at the parietal cells is ACh. The mediator at the gastrin cell is **gastrin-releasing peptide** (GRP) **or bombesin**. The direct effect on the parietal cell is the more important in humans, for selective vagotomy of the parietal cell–containing area of the stomach abolishes the response to sham-feeding, whereas antrectomy only moderately reduces it. The mechanisms involved in the cephalic phase are illustrated in Figure 8-7.

Gastric Phase

Acid secretion during the gastric phase accounts for at least 50% of the response to a meal. When swallowed food first enters the stomach and mixes with the small volume of juice normally present, buffers (primarily protein) contained in the food neutralize the acid. The pH of the gastric contents may rise to 6 or above. Because gastrin release is inhibited when the antral pH drops below 3 and is prevented totally when the pH is less than 2, essentially no gastrin is released from the stomach that is void of food. The rise in pH permits vagal stimulation from the cephalic phase to initiate, and stimuli from the gastric phase to maintain, gastrin release. It is important to realize that increasing the pH of the gastric contents is not, in itself, a stimulus for gastrin release but merely allows other stimuli to be effective.

Distention of the stomach and bathing the gastric mucosa with certain chemicals, primarily amino acids and peptides, are the effective stimuli of the gastric phase. Distention activates mechanoreceptors in the mucosa of both the oxyntic and the pyloric gland areas. It also may activate long extramural reflexes or local short intramural reflexes. All distention reflexes are mediated cholinergically and can be blocked by atropine.

Long reflexes also are called **vagovagal reflexes**, meaning that both afferent impulses and efferent impulses are carried by neurons in the vagus nerve. Mucosal distention receptors send signals by vagal afferents to the vagal nucleus. Efferent signals are sent back to G cells and parietal cells by the vagal efferents.

Short or local reflexes are mediated by neurons that are contained entirely within the wall of the stomach. These may be single-neuron reflexes, or they may involve intermediary neurons. There are two local distention reflexes. Both of these are regional reflexes, meaning that the receptor and effector are located in the same area of the stomach. Distention of a vagally innervated pyloric (antrum) pouch stimulates gastrin release. The effect is decreased, but not abolished, by vagotomy—meaning that the gastrin response is mediated by both vagovagal reflexes and local reflexes. This local reflex is called a pyloropyloric reflex.

Distention of an antral pouch with pH 1 hydrochloric acid stimulates acid secretion from the oxyntic gland area. Because gastrin release does not take place when the pH is below 2, the increase in acid output must be mediated by a neural reflex. As the discerning reader will have surmised, this vagovagal reflex is known as a *pylorooxyntic reflex*. Distention reflexes, which are much more effective stimulants of the parietal cell than they are of the G cell, are illustrated diagrammatically in Figure 8-8.

Peptides and amino acids stimulate gastrin release from the G cells. This effect is not blocked by vagotomy. Only part of it appears to be blocked by atropine, indicating that protein digestion products contain chemicals capable of directly stimulating the G cell to release gastrin. Acidification of the antral mucosa below pH 3 inhibits gastrin release in response to digested protein. A few other commonly ingested substances are also capable of stimulating acid secretion. Caffeine stimulates the parietal cells directly. Calcium, either in the gastric lumen or as elevated serum concentrations, stimulates gastrin release and acid secretion. Considerable debate exists about the effects of alcohol on gastric secretion. Alcohol has been shown to stimulate gastrin release and acid secretion in some species; however, these effects do not appear to take place in humans.

Release of Gastrin

Considerable evidence has accumulated favoring a mechanism similar to that in Figure 8-9 to explain the regulation of gastrin release. GRP acts on the G cell to stimulate gastrin release, and **somatostatin** acts on the G cell to inhibit release. GRP is a neurocrine released by vagal stimulation. This explains why atropine does not block vagally mediated gastrin release. Somatostatin

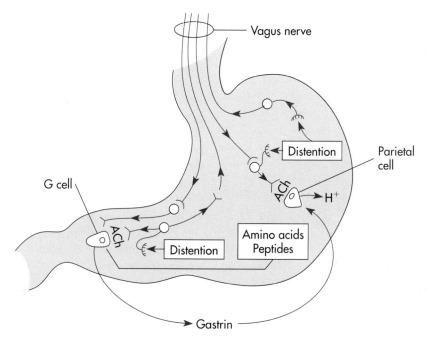

Figure 8-8 ■ Mechanisms stimulating gastric acid secretion during the gastric phase.

acts as a paracrine and its release is inhibited by vagal stimulation. In the isolated, perfused rat stomach, vagal stimulation increases GRP release and decreases somatostatin release into the perfusate. Thus it appears that vagal activation stimulates gastrin by releasing GRP and by inhibiting the release of somatostatin. Acid in the lumen of the stomach is believed to act directly on the somatostatin cell to stimulate the release of somatostatin, thereby preventing gastrin release. Protein digestion products—peptides, amino acids, and amines—may act directly on the G cell (or be absorbed by the G cell) to stimulate gastrin release.

There are data indicating that atropine can block some gastrin release stimulated by protein digestion products. This is evidence that luminal receptors may be activated, resulting in a cholinergic reflex that leads to gastrin release. There is also evidence that this reflex may operate by releasing GRP and inhibiting somatostatin release. Much of the foregoing is not proved, but the student should be familiar with the major components of this mechanism.

Intestinal Phase

Protein digestion products in the duodenum stimulate acid secretion from denervated gastric mucosa, indicating the presence of a hormonal mechanism. In humans, the proximal duodenum is rich in gastrin, which has been shown to contribute to the serum gastrin response to a meal. In dogs, liver extract releases a hormone from the duodenal mucosa that stimulates acid secretion without increasing serum gastrin levels. This hormone tentatively has been named *enterooxyntin*. Its significance in humans is unknown.

Intravenous infusion of amino acids has recently been shown to stimulate acid secretion. Therefore a good portion of the stimulation at-

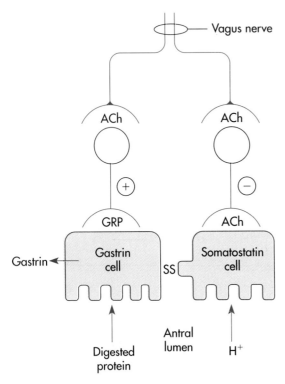

Figure 8-9 ■ Mechanism for the regulation of gastrin release.

tributed to the intestinal phase may be caused by absorbed amino acids. Intestinal stimuli result in only about 5% of the acid response to a meal. The gastric phase is responsible for most acid secretion.

Figure 8-10 summarizes the mechanisms and final stimulants acting in all three phases.

■ INHIBITION OF ACID SECRETION

When food first enters the stomach, its buffers neutralize the small volume of gastric acid present during the interdigestive phase. As the pH of the antral mucosa rises above 3, gastrin is released by the stimuli of the cephalic and gastric phases. One hour after the meal, the rate of gastric secretion is maximal, the buffering capacity of the meal is saturated, a significant portion of

the meal has emptied from the stomach, and the acid concentration of the gastric contents increases. As the pH falls, gastrin release is inhibited, removing a significant factor for the stimulation of gastric acid secretion. This passive negative feedback mechanism is extremely important in the regulation of acid secretion. In addition, somatostatin released by the drop in intragastric pH also directly inhibits the parietal cells.

Evidence exists for several hormonal mechanisms for the active inhibition of gastric acid secretion. These hormones are released from duodenal mucosa by acid, fatty acids, or hyperosmotic solutions and collectively are termed **enterogastrones**. They often inhibit gastric emptying as well as acid secretion. Teleologically these mechanisms ensure that the gastric contents are delivered to the small bowel at a rate that does not exceed the capacity for digestion and absorption. They also prevent damage to the duodenal mucosa that can result from acidic and hyperosmotic solutions.

Gastric inhibitory peptide (GIP) is released by fatty acids and acts at the parietal cell to inhibit acid secretion. **Secretin** also may be classified as an enterogastrone because it also inhibits gastric acid secretion. The importance and physiologic significance of these effects in humans have not been determined. **Cholecystokinin** is a physiologically significant inhibitor of gastric emptying. Hyperosmotic solutions release an as yet unidentified enterogastrone. Strong evidence also exists that acid initiates a nervous reflex from receptors in the duodenal mucosa that suppresses acid secretion. These mechanisms are summarized in Figure 8-11.

■ PEPSIN

Pepsinogen has a molecular weight of 42,500 and is split to form the active enzyme pepsin, which has a molecular weight of 35,000. Pepsinogen is converted to pepsin in the gastric

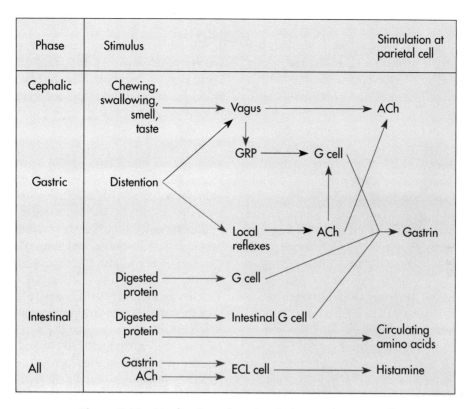

Figure 8-10 ■ **Mechanisms for stimulating acid secretion.**

Region	Stimulus	Mediator	Inhibit gastrin release	Inhibit acid secretion
Antrum	Acid (pH <3.0)	Somatostatin	+	+
Duodenum	Acid	Secretin	+	+
		Nervous reflex		+
	Hyperosmotic solutions	Unidentified enterogastrone		+
Duodenum and jejunum	Fatty acids	GIP	+	+
		Unidentified enterogastrone		+

Figure 8-11 ■ **Mechanisms for inhibiting acid secretion.**

juice when the pH drops below 5. Pepsin itself can catalyze the formation of additional pepsin from pepsinogen. Pepsin begins the digestion of protein by splitting interior peptide linkages. (See Chapter 11.)

Pepsinogens belong to two main groups, I and II. Those in the first group are secreted by peptic and mucous cells of the oxyntic glands; those in the second, by mucous cells present in the pyloric gland area and duodenum, as well as in the oxyntic gland area. Pepsinogens appear in the blood, and there is considerable evidence that their levels may be correlated with duodenal ulcer formation. This is discussed in connection with peptic ulcer disease (p. 86).

The strongest stimulant of pepsinogen secretion is ACh. Thus vagal activation during both cephalic and gastric phases results in a significant proportion of the total pepsinogen secreted. Hydrogen ion plays an important role in several areas of pepsin physiology. First, acid is necessary to convert pepsinogen to the active enzyme pepsin. At pH 2 this conversion is almost instantaneous. Second, acid triggers a local cholinergic reflex that stimulates the chief cells to secrete. This mechanism is atropine sensitive and may account in part for the strong correlation between acid and pepsin outputs. Third, the acid-sensitive reflex greatly enhances the effects of other stimuli on the peptic cell. This mechanism ensures that large amounts of pepsinogen are not secreted unless sufficient acid for conversion to pepsin is present. Fourth, acid releases the hormone secretin from duodenal mucosa. Secretin also stimulates pepsinogen secretion, although it is questionable whether enough secretin is present to do so under normal conditions.

The hormone gastrin usually is listed as a pepsigogue. Infusion of gastrin increases pepsin secretion. In dogs, the entire response can be accounted for by the stimulation of acid secretion by gastrin and the subsequent activation of the acid-sensitive reflex mechanism for pepsinogen secretion. In humans, gastrin may be a weak pepsigogue in its own right. The mechanisms regulating pepsinogen secretion are summarized in Figure 8-12.

■ MUCUS

Vagal nerve stimulation and ACh increase soluble mucus secretion from the mucous neck cells. Soluble mucus consists of mucoproteins and mixes with the gastric chyme lubricating it.

Surface mucous cells secrete visible or insoluble mucus in response to chemical stimulants (such as ethanol) and in response to physical contact and friction with roughage in the diet. Visible mucus is secreted as a gel that entraps the alkaline component of the surface cell secretion. It is present during the interdigestive phase and protects the mucosa with an alkaline layer of lubricant. A portion of this coating is made up of mucus-containing surface cells that have been shed and trapped in the layer of mucus. During the response to a meal, insoluble mucus protects the mucosa from physical and chemical damage. It neutralizes a certain amount of acid and prevents pepsin from coming into contact with the mucosa. On contact with acid, insoluble mucus precipitates into clumps and passes into the duodenum with the chyme.

■ INTRINSIC FACTOR

Intrinsic factor is a mucoprotein with a molecular weight of 55,000 secreted by the parietal cells. It combines with vitamin B_{12} in the stomach, forming a complex that is necessary for the absorption of this vitamin by the ileal mucosa. Failure to secrete intrinsic factor is associated with achlorhydria and the absence of parietal cells, which results in vitamin B_{12} deficiency or pernicious anemia. The development of this disease is poorly understood, for the liver stores enough vitamin B_{12} to last several years. The disease therefore is not recognized until long after

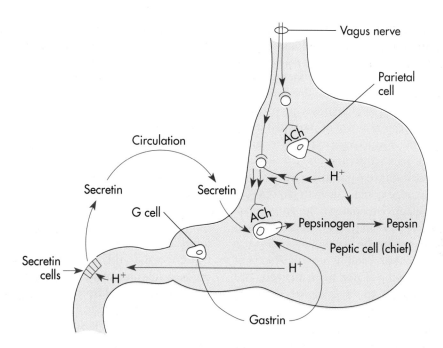

Figure 8-12 ■ Summary of mechanisms for stimulating pepsinogen secretion and activation to pepsin.

the changes have taken place in the gastric mucosa.

■ GROWTH OF THE MUCOSA

The growth of the GI mucosa is influenced by non-GI hormones and factors associated with the ingestion and digestion of a meal, such as GI hormones, nervous stimulation, secretions, and trophic substances present in the diet. Hypophysectomy results in atrophy of the digestive tract mucosa and the pancreas. The effects of hypophysectomy on growth can be prevented by administration of growth hormone. When administered to hypophysectomized rats, gastrin prevents atrophy of the GI mucosa and exocrine pancreas but does not affect the growth of other tissues. There is interesting evidence that adrenocortical steroids may trigger early postnatal development of the GI tract.

Gastrin is an important and necessary regulator of the growth of the oxyntic gland mucosa. It also stimulates growth of the intestinal and colonic mucosa and the exocrine pancreas. In humans, antrectomy causes atrophy of the remaining gastric mucosa; in rats, it causes atrophy of all GI mucosa (except that of the antrum and esophagus) and the exocrine pancreas. These changes are prevented by administration of exogenous gastrin. Hypergastrinemia results primarily in an increase in parietal and ECL cells. Gastrin is a potent stimulator of ECL-cell proliferation, and prolonged hypergastrinemia leads to ECL-cell hyperplasia.

Partial resection of the small intestine for tumor removal or for a variety of other reasons (such as treatment of morbid obesity) results in adaptation of the remaining mucosa. The mucosa of the entire digestive tract undergoes hyperplasia, which increases its ability to digest and transport nutrients or, in the case of the stomach, to secrete acid. Resection increases gastrin levels but not sufficiently to account for the adaptive changes. There is evidence that increased exposure of the mucosa to luminal contents plays an important role. After removal of proximal intestine, the distal intact mucosa is exposed to an increased load of pancreatic juice, bile, and nutrients. Investigators have hypothesized that bile and pancreatic juice contain growth factors that stimulate the adaptive response. The growth factors have not been isolated and tested. Increased uptake of nutrients by the distal mucosa also has been hypothesized to result in growth. Effects of specific nutrients have not been proved, and there is disagreement whether growth is caused by an increased work load or the increase in the available supply of calories. Good evidence exists that a hormone different from gastrin also is involved in the adaptive response.

The diet also contains polyamines that are required for growth. Trophic agents like gastrin stimulate polyamine synthesis in the proliferative cells. Thus increased luminal polyamines from the diet, coupled with synthesis stimulated by trophic hormones, may explain the regulation of mucosal growth triggered by changes in the diet.

■ PATHOPHYSIOLOGY

Gastric and duodenal ulcers are lumped together under the heading of peptic ulcer disease. Although formation of both types of ulcer requires acid and pepsin, their etiologies are basically different. Quite simply, an ulcer forms when damage by acid and pepsin overcomes the ability of the mucosa to protect itself and replace damaged cells. In the case of gastric ulcer the defect more often is in the ability of the mucosa to withstand injury. In the case of duodenal ulcer there is good evidence that the mucosa is exposed to increased amounts of acid and pepsin. This analysis is an oversimplification, for both factors no doubt are important in all cases of ulcer.

Representative acid secretory rates for normal individuals and patients with GI disorders are shown in Table 8-1. Maximal acid secretory output sometimes is measured but, in itself, is of little value in diagnosing ulcer disease. Normal subjects secrete approximately 25 mEq H^+/hr, in response to maximal injection of histamine, betazole, or gastrin. The mean output of patients

---

T A B L E   8 - 1

Comparison of acid output values from the human stomach*

Condition	Representative ranges	
	Basal acid output (mEq/hr)	Maximal acid output (mEq/hr)
Normal	1 to 5	6 to 40
Gastric ulcer	0 to 3	1 to 20
Pernicious anemia	0	0 to 10
Duodenal ulcer	2 to 10	15 to 60
Zollinger-Ellison syndrome (gastrinoma)	10 to 30	30 to 80

*Basal acid output occurs at rest, and maximal acid output during stimulation with histamine. The value is determined by multiplying the hourly volume of gastric juice aspirated times the hydrogen ion concentration of the juice.

with duodenal ulcer disease is approximately 40 mEq H⁺/hr, but the degree of overlap between individuals is so great as to render the determination useless in diagnosis. The highest rates of acid secretion are seen in cases of gastrinoma (Zollinger-Ellison syndrome), but again individual overlap makes it impossible to differentiate between this condition and duodenal ulcer on the basis of secretory data alone. Lower than normal secretory rates are found in cases of gastric ulcer, and still lower secretory rates are found in patients with gastric carcinoma. Many patients in the latter two groups, however, fall well within the normal range.

Because of the feedback mechanism whereby antral acidification inhibits gastrin release, the general statement can be made that serum gastrin levels are related inversely to acid secretory capacity. Patients with gastric ulcer and carcinoma usually have higher than normal serum gastrin levels. Serum gastrin levels in pernicious anemia actually may approach those seen in gastrinoma. Obviously, gastrinoma patients are an exception to this rule because their hypergastrinemia is derived not from the antrum but from a tumor not subject to inhibition by gastric acid. Except for the special tests mentioned in Chapter 1, serum gastrin levels cannot be used to differentiate various secretory abnormalities.

The decreased rate of acid secretion in gastric ulcer is caused in part by the failure to recover acid that has been secreted and then has leaked back across the damaged gastric mucosa. The concept of the gastric mucosal barrier is illustrated in Figure 8-13. The normal gastric mucosa is relatively impermeable to H⁺. If the gastric mucosal barrier is weakened or damaged, H⁺ leaks into the mucosa in exchange for Na⁺. As H⁺ accumulates in the mucosa, intracellular buffers are saturated and pH of the cells decreases, resulting in injury and cell death. Potassium leaks from the damaged cells into the lumen. Hydrogen ion damages mucosal mast cells. They then release histamine, which exacerbates the condition by acting on the mucosal capillaries. The result is local ischemia, hypoxia, and vascular stasis. Plasma proteins and pepsin leak into the gastric juice; and if damage is severe, bleeding occurs. Common agents that produce mucosal damage of this type are aspirin, ethanol, and bile salts. The mucosal lesions produced by topical damage to the gastric barrier may be forerunners of gastric ulcer.

The exact nature of the barrier is unknown. It is probably physiologic as well as anatomic. Cell membranes and junctional complexes prevent normal back-diffusion of H⁺. Diffused H⁺ normally is transported actively back into the lumen.

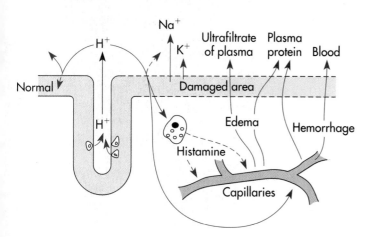

Figure 8-13 ■ Events that follow damage to the gastric mucosal barrier.

Factors that have been speculated to play a role in maintaining mucosal resistance are blood flow, mucus, cellular renewal, and chemical factors such as gastrin, prostaglandins, and epidermal growth factor. The last three agents have all been shown to decrease the severity and promote the healing of gastric ulcers.

Factors that have been elucidated as important in duodenal ulcer formation pertain to acid and pepsin secretion. Duodenal ulcer patients have on the average 2 billion parietal cells and can secrete about 40 mEq H^+/hr. Comparable measurements for normal individuals are about 50% of this. In addition, the secretion of pepsin is doubled in the duodenal ulcer group, as can be detected by measuring plasma pepsinogen. Although fasting serum gastrin is normal in patients with duodenal ulcer, the gastrin response to a meal and the sensitivity to gastrin are increased. Increased serum gastrin after a meal is caused in part by the fact that acid suppresses gastrin release less effectively in duodenal ulcer patients than in controls. The increased parietal cell mass may therefore by caused by the trophic effect of gastrin.

Work done during the last several years has established that the major acquired factor in the etiology of both gastric and duodenal ulcer is the bacterium *Helicobacter pylori*. The infection is found in 95% of patients with duodenal ulcer and virtually 100% of patients with gastric ulcers whose ulcers were not caused by chronic use of aspirin or other nonsteroidal antiinflammatory drugs (NSAIDS). *H. pylori* is a gram negative bacterium, characterized by a high urease activity, which metabolizes urea into NH_4^+. This reaction allows the bacterium to withstand the acid environment of the stomach and to colonize the mucosa. The NH_4^+ production is believed to be the major cause of cytotoxicity, for NH_4^+ directly damages epithelial cells and increases the permeability of the mucosa, i.e., "breaks the mucosal

barrier." It is also likely that the bacteria produce numerous other factors that also damage cells. All of these probably contribute to gastric ulcer formation.

H. pylori also appears to cause the increased acid secretion associated with duodenal ulcer. A recent study found that compared with normal individuals, patients with duodenal ulcer had increased basal acid output, increased GRP-stimulated acid output, increased maximal acid output in response to gastrin, increased ratio of basal acid output to gastrin-stimulated maximal acid output, and increased ratio of GRP-stimulated maximal acid output to gastrin-stimulated maximal acid output. All of these, except the increased maximal acid output in response to gastrin, totally disappeared following eradication of the *H. pylori* infection. The increased acid secretory and serum gastrin responses to GRP appear to be related to a decreased inhibition of gastrin release and parietal cell secretion by somatostatin in *H. pylori* infected individuals. While all of the mechanisms by which *H. pylori* affects the mucosa have not been elucidated, the information available appears to coincide with the known pathophysiology of both gastric and duodenal ulcer diseases.

Medical treatment of duodenal ulcer disease usually consists of administering antacids to neutralize secreted acid or a histamine H_2-receptor blocker to inhibit secretion. The H^+, K^+-ATPase (H^+ pump) inhibitor, omeprazole, blocks all acid secretion. It is extremely effective in treating duodenal ulcers—even those caused by gastrinoma. Surgical treatment is based entirely on physiology. The most commonly used operations are vagotomy and/or antrectomy. These procedures result in a 60% to 70% decrease in acid secretion by removing one or both major stimulants of acid secretion and their potentiating interaction. With the advent of the H_2 blockers and omeprazole, ulcers are now rarely treated by surgical intervention. To prevent recurrence, physicians also try to eradicate *H. pylori*. This is best done by giving antibiotics in combination with omeprazole, which increases the susceptibility of the bacteria to antibiotic treatment.

■ SUMMARY

1. The functions of gastric juice are attributed to acid, pepsin, intrinsic factor, and mucus.
2. Acid is secreted in concentrations as high as 150 mEq/L at high rates of secretion; and acid converts inactive pepsinogen to the active enzyme pepsin, kills bacteria, and solubilizes some foodstuffs.
3. Acid is secreted by the parietal cells, which contain the enzyme H^+, K^+-ATPase on their apical secretory membranes.
4. The concentrations of the electrolytes in gastric juice vary with the rate of secretion.
5. The three major stimulants of acid secretion are the hormone gastrin, the cholinergic neuromediator ACh, and the paracrine histamine, which is released from ECL cells in response to gastrin and ACh.
6. During the cephalic phase of secretion, vagal activation stimulates the parietal cells directly via ACh and releases gastrin from the G cells via GRP.
7. During the gastric phase of secretion distention of the wall of the stomach stimulates the parietal cells and releases gastrin via both mucosal and vagovagal reflexes, and protein digestion products stimulate the G cells directly to release gastrin.
8. When the pH of luminal contents drops below 3, somatostatin is released from D cells in the antrum and oxyntic gland area, where it inhibits gastrin release and acid secretion, respectively.
9. Acid secretion is inhibited further when chyme enters the duodenum and triggers the release of inhibitory hormones and initiates inhibitory neural reflexes.
10. Pepsinogen secretion is stimulated by vagal activation and ACh and by acid in the lumen of the stomach.
11. Intrinsic factor, secreted by the parietal cells, is required for the absorption of vitamin B_{12} by a specific carrier mechanism located in the ileum.

■ KEY WORDS AND CONCEPTS

- Intrinsic factor
- Hydrogen ion
- Pepsin
- Mucus
- Gastric mucosal barrier
- Oxyntic gland area
- Pyloric gland area
- Antrum
- Parietal cells
- Peptic or chief cells
- Pepsinogen
- Tubulovesicles
- Intracellular canaliculus
- Carbonic anhydrase
- H^+, K^+-ATPase
- Histamine
- Potentiation
- Cimetidine
- Enterochromaffin-like cells
- Gastrin-releasing peptide or bombesin
- Vagovagal reflexes
- Somatostatin
- Enterogastrones
- Gastric inhibitory peptide
- Secretin
- Cholecystokinin

■ BIBLIOGRAPHY

Beaumont W: *Experiments and observations on the gastric juice and the physiology of digestion*, New York, 1955, Dover Publishers.

El-Omar EM, Penman ID, Ardill JES, Chittajalln RS, Howie C, McColl KEL: Helicobacter pylori infection and abnormalities of acid secretion in patients with duodenal ulcer disease, *Gastroenterology* 109:681-691, 1995.

Feldman M, Richardson CT: Gastric acid secretion in humans. In Johnson LR, editor: *Physiology of the gastrointestinal tract*, New York, 1981, Raven Press.

Forte JG, Wolosin JM: HCl secretion by the gastric oxyntic cell. In Johnson LR, editor: *Physiology of the gastrointestinal tract*, ed 2, New York, 1987, Raven Press.

Hersey SJ: Gastric secretion of pepsinogens. In Johnson LR, editor: *Physiology of the gastrointestinal tract*, ed 3, New York, 1994, Raven Press.

Johnson LR, McCormack SA: Regulation of gastrointestinal growth. In Johnson LR, editor: *Physiology of the gastrointestinal tract*, ed 3, New York, 1994, Raven Press.

Lloyd KCK, Debas HT: Peripheral regulation of gastric acid secretion. In Johnson LR, editor: *Physiology of the gastrointestinal tract*, ed 3, New York, 1994, Raven Press.

Robert A, Nezamis JE, Lancaster C, Hanchar AJ: Cytoprotection by prostaglandins in rats. Prevention of gastric necrosis produced by alcohol, HCl, NaOH, hypertonic NaCl, and thermal injury, *Gastroenterology* 77:433-443, 1979.

Sachs G: The gastric H, K ATPase: Regulation and structure/function of the acid pump of the stomach. In Johnson LR, editor: *Physiology of the gastrointestinal tract*, ed 3, New York, 1994, Raven Press.

Saffouri B, DuVal JW, Makhlouf GM: Stimulation of gastrin secretion in vitro by intraluminal chemicals: regulation by intramural cholinergic and noncholinergic neurons, *Gastroenterology* 87:557-561, 1984.

Silen W: Gastric mucosal defense and repair. In Johnson LR, editor: *Physiology of the gastrointestinal tract*, ed 2, New York, 1987, Raven Press.

Pancreatic Secretion

Leonard R. Johnson

ancreatic exocrine secretion is divided conveniently into an aqueous or bicarbonate component and an enzymatic component. The function of the **aqueous component** is the neutralization of the duodenal contents. As such, it prevents damage to the duodenal mucosa by acid and pepsin and brings the pH of the contents into the optimum range for activity of the pancreatic enzymes. The **enzymatic or protein component** is a low-volume secretion containing enzymes for the digestion of all normal constituents of a meal. Unlike the enzymes secreted by the stomach and salivary glands, the pancreatic enzymes are essential to normal digestion and absorption.

■ FUNCTIONAL ANATOMY

The exocrine pancreas can best be likened to a cluster of grapes, and its functional units resemble the salivons of the salivary glands. Groups of acini form lobules separated by areolar tissue. Each acinus is formed from several pyramidal **acinar cells** oriented with their apices toward the lumen. The lumen of the spherical acinus is drained by a ductule whose epithelium extends into the acinus in the form of centroacinar cells. Ductules join to form intralobular ducts, which

in turn drain into interlobular ducts. These join the major pancreatic duct draining the gland.

The acinar cells secrete a small volume of juice rich in protein. Essentially all the proteins present in pancreatic juice are digestive enzymes. **Ductule cells** and **centroacinar cells** produce a large volume of watery secretion containing Na^+ and HCO_3^- as its major constituents.

Distributed throughout the pancreatic parenchyma are the **islets of Langerhans** or the endocrine pancreas. The islets produce insulin from the β cells and glucagon from the α cells. In addition, the pancreas produces the candidate hormone, pancreatic polypeptide, and contains large amounts of somatostatin, which may act as a paracrine to inhibit the release of insulin and glucagon.

The efferent nerve supply to the pancreas includes both sympathetics and parasympathetics. Sympathetic postganglionic fibers emanate from the celiac and superior mesenteric plexuses and accompany the arteries to the organ. Parasympathetic preganglionic fibers are distributed by branches of the vagi coursing down the antralduodenal region. Hence, surgical vagotomy for peptic ulcer disease affects not only the intended target organ, the hypersecreting stomach, but also the pancreas. Recently more selective operations have been designed to resect only the vagal branches passing to the stomach. Vagal fibers terminate at either acini and islets or intrinsic cholinergic nerves of the pancreas. In general the sympathetic nerves inhibit, and the parasympathetic nerves stimulate, pancreatic exocrine secretion.

■ MECHANISMS OF FLUID AND ELECTROLYTE SECRETION

The pancreas secretes approximately 1 L of fluid per day. At all rates of secretion, pancreatic juice is essentially isotonic with extracellular fluid. At low rates the primary ions are Na^+ and Cl^-. At high rates Na^+ and HCO_3^- predominate. Potassium ions are present at all rates of secretion at a concentration equal to their concentration in plasma. The concentrations of Na^+ in pancreatic juice and plasma are also approximately equal.

The aqueous component is secreted by the ductule and centroacinar cells and may contain 120 to 140 mEq HCO_3^-/L, several times its concentration in plasma. The electropotential difference across the ductule epithelium is 5 to 9 mV, lumen negative. Hence HCO_3^- is secreted against both electrical and chemical gradients. This is often considered evidence that HCO_3^- is transported actively across the luminal surface of the cells. Although the exact mechanism involved in pancreatic HCO_3^- secretion is unknown, a current model is shown in Figure 9-1. This model is based on information that shows the following: (1) over 90% of HCO_3^- in pancreatic juice is derived from plasma; (2) the secretion of HCO_3^- occurs against an electrochemical gradient and is an active process; (3) HCO_3^- secretion is blocked by ouabain, meaning that the Na^+, K^+-ATPase is involved; (4) secretion involves Na^+-H^+ and Cl^--HCO_3^- exchangers and carbonic anhydrase; and (5) HCO_3^- secretion is decreased significantly in the absence of extracellular Cl^-.

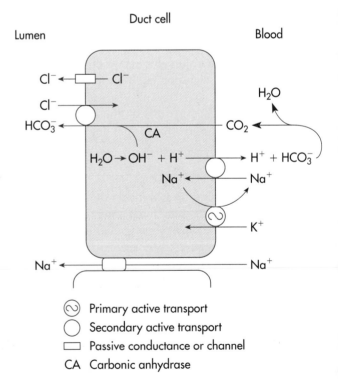

Figure 9-1 ■ Model for the secretion of HCO_3^- by the pancreatic duct cell.

The initial step in Figure 9-1 is the diffusion of CO_2 into the cell, its hydration by carbonic anhydrase and dissociation into H^+ and HCO_3^-. The H^+ is transported across the basolateral membrane either by the Na^+-H^+ exchanger or a H^+-ATPase. This is the active step in the process and results in the accumulation of HCO_3^- in the cytoplasm. The step either depends on the Na^+ gradient established by the Na^+, K^+-ATPase or the pumping of H^+ by an H^+-ATPase. In either case, the cell is alkalinized allowing more CO_2 to diffuse in. The HCO_3^- moves across the apical membrane in exchange for Cl^-. When H^+ reaches the plasma it combines with HCO_3^- to produce additional CO_2. The rate of HCO_3^- secretion depends on the availability of luminal Cl^-, which is dependent on the opening of the Cl^- channel in the apical membrane. This channel is activated by cyclic adenosine monophosphate (cAMP) in response to stimulation by secretin and is present in duct but not acinar cells. Na^+ moves down the established electrochemical gradient from the plasma to the lumen of the gland. Water passively moves from the plasma across the cells into the lumen, down the osmotic gradient created by the secretion of Na^+ and HCO_3^-. This secretion is similar to that occurring in the parietal cells of the stomach, except that the H^+ and HCO_3^- are transported in opposite directions. Thus the venous blood from an actively secreting pancreas has a lower pH than that from an inactive gland.

As in gastric juice the ionic concentrations in pancreatic juice vary with the rates of secretion (Figure 9-2). The concentrations of anions (Cl^- and HCO_3^-) in pancreatic juice are related in-

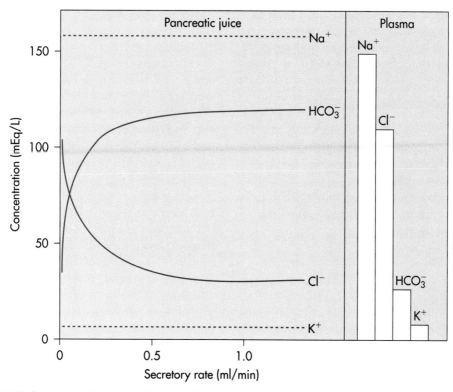

Figure 9-2 ■ **Relationship between the rate of secretion of pancreatic juice and the concentrations of its major ions.**

versely to each other, as are the concentrations of cations (Na^+ and H^+) in gastric juice. Because these relationships are analogous it might be surmised that analogous theories have been proposed to explain them.

- The two-component hypothesis assumes that one cell type, the acinar cell, secretes a small amount of fluid whose major ions are Na^+ and Cl^-. The duct cells secrete large volumes of juice rich in Na^+ and HCO_3^- in response to stimulation. At low rates of secretion, the Cl^- concentration of the juice is therefore relatively high. As the secretory rate increases, the fixed amount of Cl^- being secreted is diluted by the much larger volume of HCO_3^- -containing juice, and the final concentrations of the two anions approach the pure HCO_3^- secretion.

- Another theory proposes that the cells primarily secrete HCO_3^- and that, as it moves down the ducts, it is exchanged for Cl^-. At low rates of secretion there is sufficient time for exchange to be nearly complete, and the concentration of each anion is equal to its concentration in plasma. As the rate of secretion increases, less time is available for exchange, and the final ionic makeup of pancreatic juice approaches that of the originally secreted solution containing only HCO_3^- and Na^+. Both processes are probably involved in determining the final makeup of the secreted juice.

■ MECHANISMS OF ENZYME SECRETION

The pancreatic acinar cells synthesize and secrete major enzymes for the digestion of all three primary foodstuffs. Like pepsin, the pancreatic proteases are secreted as inactive enzyme precursors and are converted to active forms in the lumen. Pancreatic amylase and lipase are secreted in active forms. The activation and specific actions of the pancreatic enzymes are covered in detail in Chapter 11.

Although a certain amount of controversy exists concerning the mechanisms involved in the synthesis and secretion of enzymes by the acinar cells, the process outlined in Figure 9-3 is accepted by most authorities. The secretory process begins with the synthesis of exportable proteins in association with polysomes attached to the cisternae of the rough endoplasmic reticulum (RER) (step *1*). As it is being synthesized the elongating protein, directed by a leader sequence of hydrophobic amino acids, enters the cisternal cavity, where it is collected after synthesis has become complete (step *2*). Once within the cisternal space, enzymes remain membrane-bound until they are secreted from the cell. The enzymes next move through the cisternae of the RER to transitional elements, which are associated with smooth vesicles at the Golgi periphery. Possibly as a result of pinching off the transitional elements containing them, the enzymes become associated with the Golgi vesicles (step *3*), which transport them to condensing vacuoles (step *4*). Energy is required for the transport through the endoplasmic reticulum and Golgi vesicles to the condensing vacuoles. Within the condensing vacuoles the enzymes are concentrated to form zymogen granules (step *5*). They then are stored in the zymogen granules that collect at the apex of the cell. After a secretory stimulus the membrane of the zymogen granule fuses with the cell membrane, ultimately rupturing and expelling the enzymes into the lumen (step *6*). This is the only step in the process that requires a secretory stimulus.

Pancreatic enzymes can also be secreted in the absence of zymogen granules. Enzyme secretion can be maintained at high rates from glands made void of granules by constant stimulation. The mechanism involved in this process and the

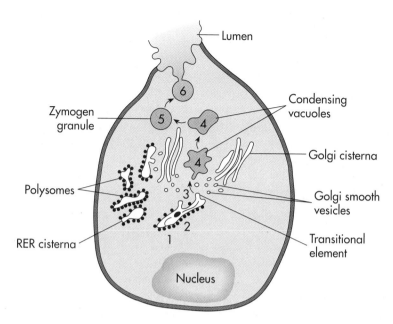

Figure 9-3 ■ **Pancreatic acinar cell. Note the major steps in the cellular synthesis and secretion of enzymes. See text for an explanation of steps 1 through 6.**

interactions between it and the zymogen granule pathway are not understood.

■ REGULATION OF SECRETION

As might be expected from its function to neutralize the duodenum, the secretion of fluid and HCO_3^- (the aqueous component) largely is determined by the amount of acid entering the duodenum. The secretion of pancreatic enzymes is, similarly, determined primarily by the amount of fat and protein entering the duodenum. Control of pancreatic secretion is regulated primarily by secretin, cholecystokinin (CCK), and vagovagal reflexes. Intestinal stimuli account for most pancreatic secretion, but secretion also is stimulated during the cephalic and gastric phases.

Basal pancreatic secretion in humans is low and difficult to measure. The basal secretion of bicarbonate is 2% to 3% of maximal, and basal enzyme secretion is 10% to 15% of maximal. The

stimuli for basal secretion are unknown. Because the isolated perfused pancreas secretes basally, this secretion may be an intrinsic property of the gland.

Cephalic Phase

Truncal vagotomy reduces the pancreatic secretory response to a meal by approximately 60%. Most of this decrease is caused by the interruption of vagovagal reflexes and by the removal of the potentiating and sensitizing effects of acetylcholine (ACh), which increase the response to secretin.

There is, however, a direct vagal component of stimulation that is initiated during the cephalic phase. Sham-feeding produces a pancreatic secretory response, which, of course, is blocked totally by vagotomy. In dogs the cephalic phase accounts for approximately 20% of the response to a meal. The stimuli for the cephalic phase of pancreatic secretion are the conditioned reflexes, smell, taste, chewing, and swallowing. Afferent impulses travel to the vagal nucleus. Vagal efferents to the pancreas stimulate both the ductule and the acinar cells to secrete. Stimulation is mediated by ACh and has a greater effect on the enzymatic component than it does on the aqueous component. In dogs a portion of the cephalic phase is mediated by gastrin released by the vagus. Gastrin has about half the potency of CCK for activating the acinar cells. Gastrin plays only a minor role, if any, in the regulation of human pancreatic secretion. These mechanisms are illustrated in Figure 9-4.

Gastric Phase

The stimulation of pancreatic secretion originating from food in the stomach is mediated by the same mechanisms that are involved in the cephalic phase. Distention of the wall of the stomach initiates vagovagal reflexes to the pancreas. Gastrin is released by protein digestion products and distention (see Chapter 8), but

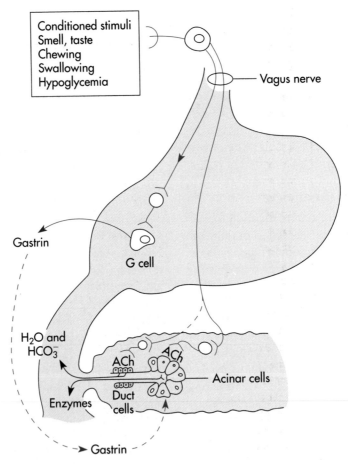

Figure 9-4 ■ **Mechanisms involved in the stimulation of pancreatic secretion during the cephalic phase. Dashed lines represent minor effects.**

again it plays little or no role in the stimulation of the human pancreas.

Intestinal Phase

The presence of digestion products and hydrogen ions in the human small intestine accounts for 70% to 80% of the stimulation of pancreatic secretion. Secretin and CCK account for almost all the hormonal stimulation of pancreatic secretion. The stimulus for the alkaline component (water and bicarbonate) is secretin released from the S cells by gastric acid and high concentrations of long-chain fatty acids. Secretion of the enzymatic component from the acinar cells is stimulated by CCK released from the I cells by fat and protein digestion products. Cholinergic reflexes also stimulate the acinar cells because vagotomy markedly reduces the enzymatic response.

The only potent releaser of secretin is hydrogen ion. The duodenal pH threshold for secretin release is 4.5. Secretin release rises almost linearly as the pH is lowered to 3 (Figure 9-5). Lowering the pH below 3 does not lead to greater release of secretin, provided the amount of titratable acid entering the duodenum is held constant. Below pH 3, secretin release and pancreatic bicarbonate secretion are related only to the amount of titratable acid entering the duodenum per unit of time. As more acid enters the gut, more secretin-containing cells are stimulated to release hormone. Thus at a constant pH the amount of secretin released is a function of the length of gut acidified. Secretin can be released from the entire duodenum and jejunum, and the amount of hormone available for release appears to be constant per centimeter of proximal small intestine.

During the response to a normal meal, however, only the duodenal bulb and proximal duodenum are acidified sufficiently to release secretin. The pH of the proximal duodenum rarely drops below 4 to 3.5. This raises doubts concerning whether sufficient secretin is released by

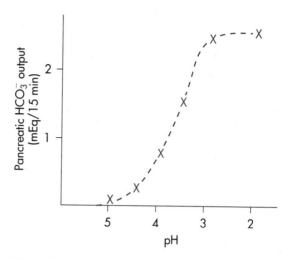

Figure 9-5 ■ Pancreatic bicarbonate output in response to various duodenal pH values. The output of bicarbonate is used as an index of secretin release.

a meal to account for the high rates of pancreatic bicarbonate and water secretion normally seen. If the pH of the gastric contents entering the duodenum is kept at 5 or higher by automatic titration, the pancreatic response is typical of CCK and ACh acting alone (a small volume of enzyme-rich juice). Dropping the pH even slightly below the threshold for secretin release leads to large increases in volume and bicarbonate secretion. The conclusion therefore is that the effects of a small amount of secretin are potentiated by CCK and ACh.

This is an important physiologic interaction of two gastrointestinal (GI) hormones and cholinergic reflexes and is demonstrated directly by the experiment outlined in Figure 9-6. Phenylalanine, a potent releaser of CCK and initiator of vagovagal reflexes, produces a small increase in volume when given alone. If, however, the same dose is infused into the gut while a low dose of secretin is given intravenously, the output of the pancreatic alkaline component increases to levels seen

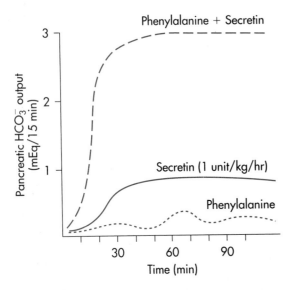

Figure 9-6 ■ **Pancreatic bicarbonate output in response to continual perfusion of the duodenum with phenylalanine, to continuous intravenous infusion of secretin, and to the combination of the two stimuli. Note that the response to secretin is greatly potentiated by endogenous phenylalanine.**

during a meal. Vagotomy greatly decreases the potentiated response. Physiologically, then, the volume and bicarbonate response to a meal result from ACh and CCK, which potentiate the effect of the small amount of secretin released by duodenal acidification.

Secretin has been referred to as "nature's antacid" because most of its physiologic and pharmacologic actions decrease the amount of acid in the duodenum. For example, it stimulates secretion of HCO_3^- from the pancreas and liver and inhibits gastric secretion and emptying as well as gastrin release.

CCK is the principal humoral stimulant of enzyme secretion from the pancreatic acinar cells. It is released in response to amino acids and fatty acids in the small intestine. Only L-isomers of amino acids are effective. In dogs, phenylalanine and tryptophan are potent releasers. Alanine, leucine, and valine are less effective. Phenylalanine, methionine, and valine appear to be potent releasers in humans. CCK is distributed evenly over the first 90 cm of intestine, and infusion of L-phenylalanine below the ligament of Treitz produces pancreatic enzyme responses equal to those seen after infusion near the pylorus. Thus the amount of CCK released depends on the load and length of bowel exposed, as well as on the concentration of amino acids present.

There is strong evidence that some peptides, as well as single amino acids, also release CCK. Three dipeptides, all of which contain glycine (*glycylphenylalanine, glycyltryptophan, phenylalanylglycine*), are effective. Dipeptides or tripeptides of glycine, or glycine itself, are ineffective. There is evidence that some peptides containing at least four amino acids are also effective. Undigested protein does not release CCK. After a protein meal, therefore, a wide variety of specific protein products evoke CCK release and pancreatic enzyme secretion.

In addition to protein products, fatty acids longer than eight carbon atoms release CCK and initiate vagovagal reflexes. *Lauric, palmitic, stearic,* and *oleic acids* are equal and strong releasers of CCK. Fat must be in an absorbable form before release of the hormone occurs. The interactions between luminal nutrients and the receptors triggering the release of CCK, and of GI hormones in general, are poorly understood. As a result, most of the intracellular mechanisms resulting in hormone release are unknown. Part of the reason for this paucity of information has been the inability to isolate large numbers of hormone-containing cells from the mucosa of the GI tract.

The mechanisms resulting in the stimulation of pancreatic secretion during the intestinal phase are illustrated in Figure 9-7.

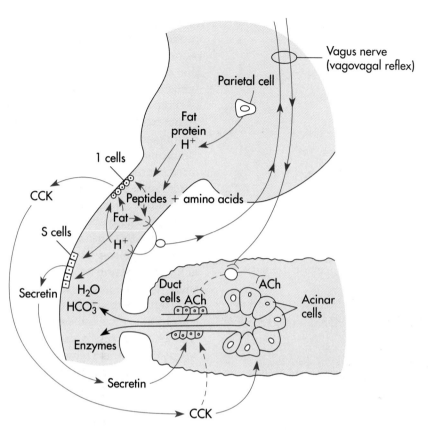

Figure 9-7 ■ Mechanisms involved in the stimulation of pancreatic secretion during the intestinal phase. Dashed lines indicate potentiative interactions with secretin.

■ CELLULAR BASIS FOR POTENTIATION

The concept of **potentiation** requires that the potentiating stimuli act on different membrane receptors and trigger different cellular mechanisms for the stimulation of secretion. Some of the steps in these mechanisms have been elucidated for the pancreatic acinar cell and are illustrated in Figure 9-8. Secretin binding to its receptor triggers an increase in adenylyl cyclase activity, resulting in the synthesis of cAMP. ACh and CCK bind to separate receptors, but both increase intracellular Ca^{++}. The Ca^{++} is mobilized primarily from the plasma membranes and rough endoplasmic reticulum of the acinar cells. Both CCK and ACh also increase diacylglycerol and inositol triphosphate production from phosphatidylinositol. It is likely that one of these breakdown products is the intracellular messenger for Ca^{++} release. Interactions between secretin and ACh or secretin and CCK result in potentiation. However, the effects of combining CCK and ACh, which trigger identical mechanisms, are only additive. Glucagon and vasoactive intestinal peptide also increase cAMP, and gas-

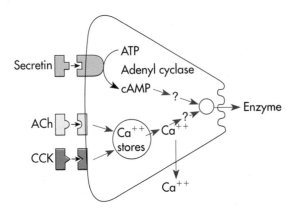

Figure 9-8 ■ Receptors on the rodent pancreatic acinar cell. Different second messengers for the stimulants indicate different cellular mechanisms for stimulation and provide the basis for potentiation.

trin, gastrin-releasing peptide, and substance P increase Ca^{++} in acinar cells. However, there is no strong evidence that these substances play an important role in the physiologic regulation of pancreatic secretion.

The final steps in the process leading to enzyme secretion have not been elucidated, but they involve the phosphorylation of structural and regulatory proteins. Potentiation occurs because Ca^{++} and cAMP phosphorylate different proteins. The foregoing interactions have been worked out with guinea pig isolated pancreatic acini. Secretin does not potentiate the effects of CCK and ACh in dogs or humans. A system similar to this, however, is a likely explanation of the potentiation in all species in which it occurs. Thus similar events may be predicted for the human ductule cell.

■ RESPONSE TO A MEAL

As digestion and mixing of food proceed in the stomach, buffers present in proteins and peptides become saturated with hydrogen ions and the pH drops to about 2. The maximum load of titratable acid (free H^+ plus bound H^+) delivered

to the duodenum is 20 to 30 mEq/hr. This is approximately equal to the maximal capacity of the stomach to secrete acid, which, in turn, equals the ability of the pancreas to secrete HCO_3^- when it is maximally stimulated. To raise the pH of the duodenum, the undissociated H^+, as well as the free H^+, must be neutralized. This is accomplished rapidly in the first part of the duodenum and the pH of the chyme is raised quickly from 2 at the pylorus to above 4 beyond the duodenal bulb. Some neutralization occurs by absorption of H^+ and secretion of bicarbonate by the gut wall. An additional amount of H^+ is neutralized by HCO_3^- in the bile. The contributions of the gut mucosa and bile, however, are small, and by far the greatest proportion of acid is neutralized by the large volume of pancreatic juice secreted into the lumen.

Within a few minutes after chyme enters the duodenum there is a sharp rise in the secretion of pancreatic enzymes. Within 30 minutes, enzyme secretion peaks at levels about 70% to 80% of those attainable with maximal stimulation by CCK and cholinergic reflexes. Enzyme secretion continues at this rate until the stomach is empty. The enzyme response to a meal may be kept below maximum by the presence of humoral inhibitors of pancreatic secretion. This is the proposed function of pancreatic polypeptide.

Pancreatic enzyme secretion is able to adapt to the diet. In other words, ingestion of a high protein, low carbohydrate diet over several days increases the proportion of proteases and decreases the proportion of amylase in pancreatic juice. This type of response is now known to be hormonally regulated at the level of gene expression. CCK increases the expression of the genes for proteases and decreases that for amylase. Secretin and gastric inhibitory peptide increase the expression of the gene for lipase. The mechanism to increase amylase gene expression under normal conditions is not known, although insulin regulates amylase levels in diabetics.

■ CLINICAL APPLICATIONS

Abnormal pancreatic secretion occurs in diseases such as chronic and acute pancreatitis, cystic fibrosis, and kwashiorkor, and in tumors that involve the gland itself. Changes in secretion during one of these diseases depend upon the stage of development of the disease. Most patients with **chronic pancreatitis** have decreased volume and bicarbonate output, whereas those with acute pancreatitis often have normal secretion. Both volume and enzyme content of pancreatic juice are decreased by cystic fibrosis. **Tumors of the pancreas** frequently decrease the volume of secretion. In **kwashiorkor,** the alkaline and enzymatic components are depressed, but amylase secretion continues after trypsin, chymotrypsin, and lipase activities are no longer found.

Cystic fibrosis is characterized by decreased Cl^- secretion of many epithelial tissues, and by the inability of cAMP to regulate Cl^- conductance. As mentioned earlier, there is good evidence that the ion channel for Cl^- in the apical membrane of the duct cell is the cystic fibrosis transmembrane conductance regulator that is regulated by cAMP. Failure to synthesize this protein in its normal state results in cystic fibrosis and a severe decrease of ductal secretion. As a result, proteinaceous acinar secretions become concentrated and precipitate within the duct lumen, blocking small ducts and eventually destroying the gland.

Pancreatic enzyme secretion must be reduced by more than 80% to produce **steatorrhea.** If a patient has steatorrhea, it is only necessary to measure the concentration of any pancreatic enzyme in the jejunal content after a meal to determine whether the condition is pancreatic in origin.

Pancreatic exocrine function is assessed by measuring basal secretion and secretion stimulated by secretin and/or CCK. These function tests are performed on a fasting patient. A double-lumen nasogastric tube is used. One tube opens into the stomach to drain gastric contents that would otherwise empty into the duodenum; the other collects duodenal juice that is assumed to be largely pancreatic in origin. Interpretation of the test is impeded by contaminating biliary secretions. Changes in secretion depend upon the stage of development of various diseases and may vary from patient to patient. For these reasons, pancreatic function tests are not reliable in the diagnosis of individual diseases but are used to assess overall pancreatic function.

■ SUMMARY

1. Pancreatic secretion consists of an aqueous bicarbonate component from the duct cells and an enzymatic component from the acinar cells.

2. The duct cells actively secrete HCO_3^- into the lumen, and Na^+ and H_2O follow down electrical and osmotic gradients respectively.

3. The composition of pancreatic juice varies with the rate of secretion. At low rates Na^+ and Cl^- predominate, and at high rates Na^+ and HCO_3^- predominate.

4. Pancreatic enzymes are essential for the digestion of all major foodstuffs and are stored in zymogen granules of acinar cells before secretion.

5. The primary stimulant of the aqueous component is secretin, whose effects are potentiated by CCK and ACh.

6. During the cephalic phase of secretion, vagal stimulation results in a low volume of secretion containing a high concentration of enzymes. This secretion is produced by the acinar cells.

7. During the intestinal phase, acid (pH <4.5) releases secretin; and acid, fats and amino acids trigger vagovagal reflexes, while fats and amino acids release CCK. CCK and ACh stimulate enzyme secretion from the acinar cells. Stimulants using different second messengers potentiate each other.

■ KEY WORDS AND CONCEPTS

- Aqueous component of pancreatic exocrine secretion
- Enzymatic or protein component of pancreatic exocrine secretion
- Acinar cells
- Ductule cells
- Centroacinar cells
- Islets of Langerhans
- Secretin
- Cholecystokinin
- Potentiation
- Chronic pancreatitis
- Tumors of the pancreas
- Kwashiorkor
- Steatorrhea
- Cystic fibrosis

■ BIBLIOGRAPHY

Anagostides A, Chadwick VS, Selden AC, Maton PN: Sham feeding and pancreatic secretion; evidence for direct vagal stimulation of enzyme output, *Gastroenterology* 87:109-114, 1984.

Argent BE, Case RM: Pancreatic ducts: cellular mechanism and control of bicarbonate secretion. In Johnson LR, editor: *Physiology of the gastrointestinal tract,* ed 3, New York, 1994, Raven Press.

Gorelick FS, Jamieson JD: The pancreatic acinar cell: structure-function relationships. In Johnson LR, editor: *Physiology of the gastrointestinal tract,* ed 3, New York, 1994, Raven Press.

Jensen RT: Receptors on pancreatic acinar cells. In Johnson LR, editor: *Physiology of the gastrointestinal tract,* ed 3, New York, 1994, Raven Press.

Meyer JH, Kelley GA, Spingola LJ, Jones RS: Canine gut receptors mediating pancreatic responses to luminal L-amino acids, *Am J Physiol* 231:669-677, 1976.

Meyer JH, Way LW, Grossman MI: Pancreatic response to acidification of various lengths of proximal intestine in the dog, *Am J Physiol* 219:971-977, 1970.

Solomon TE: Control of exocrine pancreatic secretion. In Johnson LR, editor: *Physiology of the gastrointestinal tract,* ed 3, New York, 1994, Raven Press.

Solomon TE, Grossman MI: Effect of atropine and vagotomy on response of transplanted pancreas, *Am J Physiol* 236:E186-E190, 1979.

Yule DI, Williams JA: Stimulus-secretion coupling in the pancreatic acinus. In Johnson LR, editor: *Physiology of the gastrointestinal tract,* ed 3, New York, 1994, Raven Press.

10

Bile Production, Secretion, and Storage

Norman W. Weisbrodt

S ecretion of bile is necessary for the proper digestion and absorption of lipids. It also is required for the normal elimination of various endogenous products (e.g., cholesterol, bile pigments), as well as exogenously administered chemicals (e.g., phenothiazines and heavy metals). Bile secretion is discussed here in three parts: (1) the formation of bile by the hepatocytes and biliary ducts, (2) the storage and concentration of bile in the gallbladder, and (3) the expulsion and transport of bile from the gallbladder to the lumen of the intestine.

■ BILE FORMATION
Constituents of Bile

Bile is a complex mixture of organic and inorganic components. Taken separately, some of the components are insoluble and would precipitate out of an aqueous medium. Normally, however, bile is a homogeneous and stable solution whose stability depends upon the physical behavior and interactions of its various components.

   Bile acids are the major organic constituents of bile, accounting for approximately 50% of the solid components. Chemically they are carboxylic acids with a cyclopentanophenanthrene nucleus and a branched side chain of three to nine carbon atoms that ends in a carboxyl group (Figure 10-1). They are related structurally to cholesterol, from which they are synthesized by the liver. Several features are unique to the bile acids and account for their behavior in solution. Three-dimensionally the hydroxyl and carboxyl groups are located on one side of the molecule. The bulk of the molecule is composed of the nucleus and several methyl groups (Figure 10-1). This structure renders bile acids amphipathic, to the extent that the hydroxyl and dissociated carboxyl groups are hydrophilic and the nucleus and methyl groupings are hydrophobic. In solution the behavior of bile acids depends on their concentration. At low concentrations there is little interaction among bile acid molecules. As the concentration is increased, a point is reached where aggregation of the molecules takes place. These aggregates are called **micelles,** and the point of formation is called the **critical micellar concentration.** Hydrophobic regions of the micelles interact with one another, and the hydrophilic regions interact with the water molecules. (See Figure 11-13.)

   The most common human bile acids are cholic acid, chenodeoxycholic acid, deoxycholic acid, and lithocholic acid. These differ from one

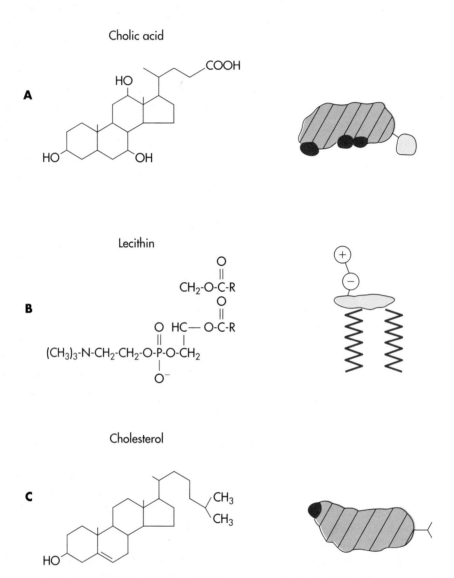

Cholic acid

A

Lecithin

B

Cholesterol

C

Figure 10-1 ■ Structural formulas for some of the components of bile. *Left,* Conventional representation; *right,* shorthand version of the Stuart-Briegleb representation. A, Cholic acid. Note that the polar hydroxyl groups *(dark circles)* and the carboxyl group are on the same side of the molecule. B, Lecithin. Note that the polar phosphatidylcholine group is at one end and the nonpolar fatty acids are at the other. C, Cholesterol. Only one hydroxyl group is present; thus cholesterol is strongly hydrophobic.

another primarily in the number of hydroxyl groups present. Cholic acid is a trihydroxy acid; deoxycholic acid and chenodeoxycholic acid are dihydroxy acids; lithocholic is a monohydroxy acid and is only slightly soluble. Another feature that affects the aqueous solubility of bile acids is the state of the terminal carboxyl group. The pK of unconjugated bile acids is near neutral; thus at the pH of intestinal contents they are mostly undissociated and relatively insoluble. In vivo, however, most bile acids exist as conjugates of taurine or glycine. Conjugated bile acids have much lower pK values and exist as the more soluble dissociated salts at pH values that are found in the biliary tract and intestine.

The second most abundant group of organic compounds in bile are the **phospholipids,** the major ones being the lecithins (Figure 10-1). Phospholipids are also amphipathic, insofar as the phosphatidylcholine grouping is hydrophilic, whereas the fatty acid chains are hydrophobic. Although amphipathic, the phospholipids are not soluble in water but form liquid crystals that swell in solution. In the presence of bile salts, however, the liquid crystals are broken up and solubilized as a component of the micelles. Bile salts possess a large capacity to solubilize phospholipids; 2 mol of lecithin are solubilized by 1 mol of bile salts. The combination of bile salts and phospholipids is also better able to solubilize other lipids—mainly cholesterol—than is a simple solution of bile salts.

A third organic component, **cholesterol,** is present in small amounts, contributing about 4% to the total solids of bile. Although present in small amounts, bile cholesterol is important since it may be excreted, and it therefore helps regulate body stores of cholesterol. Cholesterol appears mainly in the nonesterified form and is insoluble in water. In the presence of bile salts and phospholipids, however, it is solubilized as part of the micelle. Because it is a weakly polar substance, cholesterol is found in the interior of the

micelle, where the hydrophobic portions of the bile salts and phospholipids interact.

The fourth major group of organic compounds found in bile are the **bile pigments.** These constitute only 2% of the total solids, with bilirubin being the most important. Chemically, bile pigments are tetrapyrroles and are related to the porphyrins, from which they are derived. In their free form, bile pigments are insoluble in water. Normally, however, they are conjugated with glucuronic acid and rendered soluble. Unlike the other organic compounds just mentioned, bile pigments do not take part in micellar formation. As their name implies they are highly colored substances. Other than being responsible for the normal color of bile and feces, the pigment properties of these compounds are utilized to assess the level of function of the liver (pp. 110-111).

In addition to the organic compounds just discussed, many **inorganic ions** are found in bile. The predominant cation is Na^+, accompanied by smaller amounts of K^+ and Ca^{++}. The predominant inorganic anions are Cl^- and HCO_3^-. Normally the total number of inorganic cations will exceed the total number of inorganic anions. There is no anion deficit, however, because the bile acids, which possess a net negative charge at the pH values found in bile, account for the difference. Bile is isosmotic even though there is a larger than expected number of cations present. Because they are highly charged molecules, the bile acids attract a layer of cations that serve as counterions. These counterions are tightly associated with the micelles and thus exert little osmotic activity. Therefore bile is isosmotic even though there is a larger number of cations present than expected.

■ SECRETION OF BILE

The secretion of bile depends heavily upon the secretion of bile acids by the liver. Once secreted, bile acids undergo an interesting journey (Figure 10-2). First, they may be stored in the

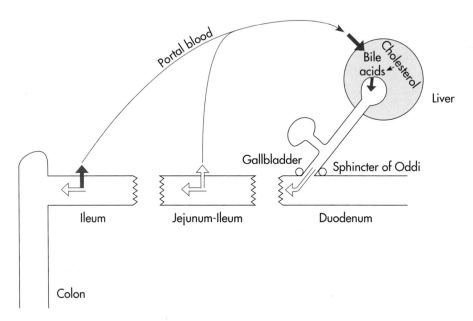

Figure 10-2 ■ Enterohepatic circulation of bile acids. Bile acids are actively secreted by the liver. Once in the intestine they participate in the digestion and absorption of lipids. As they are propelled toward the distal small bowel, some of the "primary" acids are altered, becoming "secondary" acids. The more hydrophobic bile acids are absorbed passively throughout the intestine. The more hydrophilic acids are absorbed by a sodium-coupled active transport process that is localized to the ileum. A minor fraction of bile acids is not absorbed but is propelled into the colon. The absorbed bile acids are transported via the portal circulation to the liver, where they are extracted actively from the blood (almost 100%) and resecreted. Synthesis of new primary acids from cholesterol occurs at a rate to compensate for the acids lost from the bowel. Solid arrows denote active absorption, secretion, and synthesis; open arrows denote passive absorption and propulsion of contents by contractions of the intestine.

gallbladder. Then they are propelled into and through the small intestine, where they take part in the digestion and absorption of lipids. Most of the bile acids themselves are absorbed from the intestine and travel via the portal blood to the liver, where they are taken up by the hepatocytes and resecreted. This process is termed the **enterohepatic circulation.**

Bile acids are secreted continuously by the **liver.** The rate of secretion, however, varies widely. Early experiments demonstrated that the rate of secretion depended on the amount of bile acids delivered to the liver via the blood; the more acids in the portal blood, the greater the se-

cretion of bile. The amount of bile acids in the portal blood depends upon the amount absorbed from the small intestine. The amount of bile acids in the intestine, in turn, depends upon the digestive state of the individual. Between meals, most bile secreted by the liver is stored in the gallbladder (pp. 107-109) rather than delivered to the small intestine. During a meal the gallbladder empties its contents into the duodenum in a more continuous pattern. The ejected bile acids are then resorbed from the intestine and resecreted by the liver. It is estimated that the total amount of bile acids in the body is secreted twice during the digestion of each meal.

Although a wide variety of bile acids are found in the bile, only cholic and chenodeoxycholic acids appear to be synthesized from cholesterol in significant amounts by human hepatocytes. For this reason they are called primary bile acids. Their synthesis by the liver is a continuous but regulated process. The amount synthesized depends upon the amount of bile acids returned to the liver in the enterohepatic circulation. If most of the bile acids secreted by the liver are returned, synthesis is low; but if the secreted acids are lost from the enterohepatic circulation, the rate of synthesis will be high. Normally there are 1 to 2 g of bile salts in the enterohepatic circulation. If the absorptive processes in the intestine and liver are functioning properly, only about 0.5 g is lost daily. Synthesis is regulated to replenish this loss.

Deoxycholic acid, lithocholic acid, and other "secondary" bile acids are produced in the intestine through the action of microorganisms on primary bile acids. These acids then are absorbed along with the primary bile acids, taken up by the **hepatocytes,** conjugated with taurine and glycine, and secreted in the bile. Thus bile contains a mixture of primary and secondary bile acids. Cholic, chenodeoxycholic, and deoxycholic acids normally appear in a ratio of 4:4:2. Usually only a small amount of lithocholic acid is present.

The enterohepatic circulation of bile acids is characterized by both passive and active transport processes (Figure 10-2). The more hydrophobic bile acids, those with fewer hydroxyl groups and those that become deconjugated, are absorbed passively throughout the intestine. The more hydrophilic acids are absorbed by a sodium-coupled active transport process that is localized to the ileum. As stated above, this active transport process is highly efficient. A second sodium-coupled active transport process is located within the hepatocytes. The carrier proteins mediating this process in the liver appear to differ from those found in ileal enterocytes, but appear to be just as efficient. Practically all bile acids contained in the portal blood are removed during one passage through the liver. The process does have a transport maximum, but this is seldom reached.

Cholesterol and phospholipids (primarily lecithins) also are secreted by the hepatocytes. The exact mechanisms of secretion are not known; but secretion appears to depend, in part, upon the secretion of bile acids. The higher the rate of bile acid secretion, the higher is the rate of cholesterol and phospholipid secretion. Once secreted into the intestine along with the other components of bile, cholesterol and lecithin are mixed with and handled as ingested cholesterol and lecithin (See Chapter 11.)

The primary bile pigment in humans, **bilirubin,** is derived largely from the metabolic breakdown of **hemoglobin** (Figure 10-3). Most of the hemoglobin comes from aged red blood cells that are disposed of by cells of the reticuloendothelial system. In the reticuloendothelial cells hemoglobin is split into hemin and globin. The hemin ring is opened and oxidized, and the iron is removed to form bilirubin, which is then transported via the blood from the cells of the reticuloendothelial system to the hepatocytes. In transit, bilirubin is tightly bound to plasma albumin; very little is free in the plasma. Hepatocytes possess the ability to extract bilirubin from blood, conjugate it with glucuronic acid, and secrete the conjugated product into the bile. Bilirubin uptake by the hepatocytes is mediated by an active anion transport system. This system is different from the one for active transport of bile acids, but it is shared by a number of other organic anions (e.g., sulfobromophthalein [Bromsulphalein, BSP] and various radiopaque dyes).

Bilirubin is not absorbed from the intestine in any appreciable amounts. Some of the product, however, is altered in the bowel. Bacteria, primarily in the distal small bowel and colon, re-

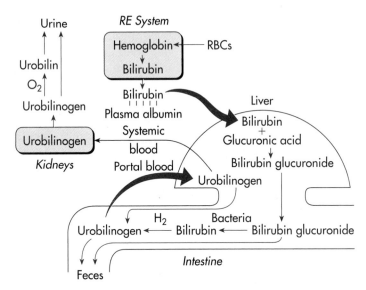

Figure 10-3 ■ **Excretion of bile pigments. Bilirubin is produced by cells of the reticuloendothelial (RE) system from aged red blood cells (RBCs). The unconjugated pigment is then carried, tightly bound to plasma albumin, to the liver. There it is actively taken up, conjugated with glucuronic acid, and secreted into the bile. The water-soluble conjugates are propelled along the intestine. In the distal small bowel and colon a portion of the conjugated pigment is acted upon by bacteria and becomes unconjugated bilirubin and other pigments. Some of these pigments are absorbed passively into the blood and either are returned to the liver and resecreted, or pass through the liver and are excreted by the kidneys. Most, however, pass through the colon and are excreted. Bold arrows indicate active absorption.**

duce bilirubin to urobilinogen, which is unconjugated. Some urobilinogen is excreted in the feces, but part is absorbed into the portal blood and returned to the liver. There most of the urobilinogen is extracted, conjugated, and secreted into the bile; however, some passes into the systemic circulation and is excreted by the kidneys. The urobilinogen is oxidized in the urine and feces to form urobilin and stercobilin, respectively. These pigments are in large part responsible for the color of the excretory products of the body.

Two components of bile water and electrolyte secretion have been identified. One is called **bile acid dependent secretion.** Bile acids, regardless of whether they are newly synthesized or extracted from the portal blood, are the major ions actively secreted by the hepatocytes. Their se-

cretion, in turn, sets up an osmotic gradient down which water moves. The movement of water is accompanied by the passive movement of electrolytes (Figure 10-4). The second component is called **bile acid independent secretion.** There is evidence for the active transport of Na^+ by the hepatocytes. Also, as the canalicular bile flows through the bile ductules and ducts on its way to the gallbladder, its composition is altered (Figure 10-4). Both secretion and absorption take place in the ducts, secretion normally predominating. Bicarbonate is actively secreted by the epithelial cells that line the ducts. Absorption of Na^+, Cl^-, and water also can be demonstrated. The net effect of this secretory and absorptive activity is that the bile becomes more alkaline and its chloride content decreases.

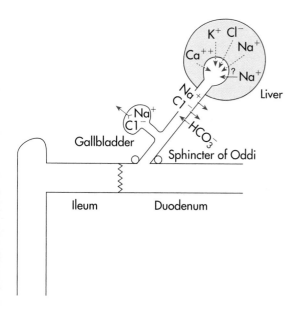

Figure 10-4 ■ Secretion and absorption of water and electrolytes. The osmotic gradient created by the active secretion of bile acids, and perhaps Na$^+$, causes water to move from the hepatocytes into the bile canaliculi. Ions accompany water movement, presumably via the process of bulk flow. Epithelial cells of the bile ducts are capable of actively absorbing Na$^+$ and Cl$^-$ and of actively secreting Na$^+$ and HCO$_3^-$. In the gallbladder, salt absorption is accompanied by the absorption of water, thus concentrating the bile.

Secretory activity of the epithelial cells of the bile ductules and ducts is under hormonal control. Secretin stimulates production of bile that is relatively low in bile salt and high in HCO$_3^-$ concentrations. It does this by increasing the active transport of sodium and bicarbonate from the epithelial cells into the bile.

■ BILE TRANSPORT TO AND STORAGE IN THE GALLBLADDER

The force responsible for flow of bile from the canaliculi toward the small intestine is primarily the secretory pressure generated by the hepatocytes and ductule epithelium. The hepatic end

of the biliary tract is blind, being formed by the secretory cells of the liver. Thus as bile is secreted by these cells, pressure in the ducts rises. The active secretion of bile acids and electrolytes can make biliary secretory pressures reach 10 to 20 mm Hg.

Whether bile flows into the duodenum or into the gallbladder depends on a balance between the resistance to filling of the gallbladder and the resistance to flow through the terminal **bile duct** and **sphincter of Oddi.** The gallbladder is a distensible muscular organ that forms a blind outpouching of the biliary tract. Its inner surface is lined with a thin layer of epithelial cells having high absorptive capacities. The sphincter of Oddi is a thickening of the circular muscle of the bile duct located at the ductal entrance into the duodenum. Although this muscle is embedded in the wall of the duodenum, it appears to be an entity separate from the duodenal musculature. Most of the time during fasting, the gallbladder is readily distensible, and the sphincter of Oddi maintains closure of the terminal bile duct. Thus bile that is secreted by the liver flows into the gallbladder (Figure 10-5, A).

The human gallbladder is not a large organ and when full can accommodate only 20 to 50 ml of fluid. During fasting, however, many times that volume of fluid may be secreted by the liver. The discrepancy between the amount of bile secreted by the liver and the amount stored in the gallbladder is accounted for by the gallbladder's ability to concentrate bile. The concentration of bile salts, bile pigments, and other large water-soluble molecules may increase 5 to 20 times as a result of water and electrolyte absorption.

Absorption of water and electrolytes is partly an active process. Na$^+$ absorption can occur against an electrochemical gradient, is a saturable process, depends upon metabolic activity, and demonstrates other characteristics of an active transport mechanism. Unlike the transport mechanisms for Na$^+$ that exist in other epithelia, how-

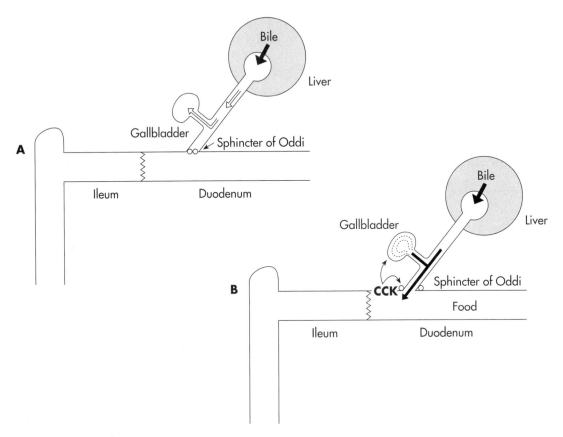

Figure 10-5 ■ A, Bile flow between periods of digestion. Bile is secreted continuously by the liver and flows toward the duodenum. In the interdigestive period the gallbladder is readily distensible and the sphincter of Oddi is contracted. Therefore bile flows into the gallbladder rather than into the duodenum. **B,** On eating, both hormonal *(CCK)* and neural stimuli cause contraction of the gallbladder and relaxation of the sphincter of Oddi. Thus bile flows into the bowel. Bile secretion by the liver increases as bile acids are returned via the enterohepatic circulation.

ever, transport in the gallbladder is not associated with generation of any measurable electrical potential difference. In addition, it is highly dependent upon the presence of either Cl^- or HCO_3^-. Thus it appears as if Na^+ transport is coupled with the transport of an anion and is electrically neutral.

As in other epithelial tissue, water movement in the gallbladder is dependent upon the active absorption of NaCl and $NaHCO_3$, and thus it is entirely passive. The rows of epithelial cells of

the mucosa have large lateral intercellular spaces near the basal membrane and possess tight junctions at their apices. Solute is transported actively from the cells into the intercellular space at the apical ends. This movement is then followed by the passive diffusion of H_2O. The movement of water molecules, however, is such that an osmotic gradient is set up in the intercellular spaces. The solution is hypertonic at the apical end and isotonic at the basal end. In the steady state, this standing osmotic gradient is maintained and accounts for the absorption of a solution with fixed osmolality. (See Figure 12-5.)

Absorption of Na^+, Cl^-, HCO_3^-, and H_2O influences the concentrations of other solutes in the bile. Ions such as K^+ and Ca^{++} become more concentrated. The concentration of micelles also increases during the absorption of water and electrolytes. The presence of micelles, which have minimal osmotic activity, permits the high concentration of electrolytes, bile salts, phospholipids, and cholesterol to be isotonic in gallbladder bile.

■ EXPULSION OF BILE AND TRANSPORT TO THE INTESTINE

Most bile secretion occurs during digestion of meals. However, significant amounts are secreted periodically during fasting in synchrony with the migrating motor complex (MMC) (p. 46). The gallbladder contracts shortly before and during the period of intense sequential duodenal contractions. Thus bile, along with other secretions, is swept aborally along the bowel by these contractions. The exact stimuli and pathways responsible for coordinating gallbladder contraction with cyclic intestinal motility are not known, but appear to involve cholinergic nerves.

Shortly after eating, the gallbladder musculature contracts rhythmically and empties gradually (Figure 10-5, B). The stimulus for its contraction appears to be primarily hormonal. Products of food digestion, particularly lipids, release **cholecystokinin** (CCK) from the mucosa of the duodenum. This hormone is carried in the blood to the gallbladder, where it stimulates the musculature to contract. CCK is a potent stimulant of gallbladder muscle and may in part act by binding to receptors located directly on smooth muscle cells. In vivo, however, much of CCK's action appears to be mediated through intrinsic cholinergic nerves. The role of other gastrointestinal hormones is less clear. Gastrin stimulates gallbladder contraction, but in doses that are well

above the physiologic range. Secretin appears to have little direct effect on the gallbladder, though it may antagonize (or prevent) the effects of CCK.

Flow of bile from the gallbladder through the common bile duct, and into the duodenum, is influenced by muscular activity of the common bile duct, the sphincter of Oddi, and the duodenum. The bile duct contains smooth muscle cells, and measurements of its contractile activity have been made in certain species. Some investigators maintain that peristaltic contractions of the duct do occur, and that these facilitate movement of bile into the duodenum. The relative importance of this mechanism is not known.

The sphincter of Oddi is a muscular ring surrounding the opening of the bile duct in the wall of the duodenum. Its relative contributions to the regulation of bile flow are sometimes difficult to assess because its own activity is influenced by the musculature of the duodenum. The sphincter can maintain closure of the bile duct independent of activity of the duodenal musculature. When the duodenum is relaxed, pressures of 12 to 30 mm Hg are needed to force fluid through a closed sphincter. However, bile flow through an open sphincter of Oddi is influenced markedly by the contractile activity of the duodenum. Bile enters an actively contracting bowel in spurts during periods of duodenal relaxation and stops during periods of contraction. The sphincter, like the muscle of the gallbladder, is controlled by the hormone CCK. In contrast to its action on the gallbladder, CCK relaxes the sphincter of Oddi and thereby allows bile to enter the duodenum.

The role of the autonomic nervous system in the control of bile flow is not clear. Stimulation of parasympathetic nerves causes an increase in bile flow and contraction of the gallbladder. Stimulation of sympathetic nerves has the opposite effect. Bile flow begins shortly after eating and may be part of the cephalic phase of digestion.

The emotional state of the individual also has been shown to influence bile flow.

■ CLINICAL APPLICATIONS

Abnormalities of bile secretion can result from functional changes in the liver, bile ducts, gallbladder, and intestine. Because many of the components of bile are synthesized and/or actively secreted by hepatocytes, metabolic abnormalities of these cells can result in decreased bile production and increased plasma levels of those constituents normally excreted in the bile (e.g., bile acids and pigments). Metabolic abnormalities more commonly result from the destruction of hepatocytes by infectious agents (e.g., viral hepatitis) and by various toxins. There are, however, several conditions characterized by genetic deficiencies in one or more of the steps of bilirubin secretion. These deficiencies also can result in **jaundice** (a visually detectable buildup of bile pigments in the blood).

Besides the rather striking changes in hepatocyte function seen with hepatocyte destruction and genetic defects, subtle changes also can produce pathologic conditions. In many individuals the quantity of bile produced by the liver may be normal, but the quality abnormal. To be stable, bile must contain certain proportions of bile salts, phospholipids, and cholesterol. If there is a relative excess of cholesterol it may precipitate to form gallstones.

Abnormalities of the bile ducts and gallbladder are usually secondary to the processes of obstruction (e.g., stones or tumor) and/or infection. **Obstruction** can result in severe pain and can lead to reflux of bile into the liver parenchyma and eventually the systemic circulation. **Bacterial infections,** often occurring secondary to stones, also can initiate and/or perpetuate stone formation. Several strains of bacteria (such as *Escherichia coli*) produce β-glucuronidase, which deconjugates conjugated bile pigments. These unconjugated pigments, which are less soluble, will then precipitate to form pigment stones or a nidus for precipitation of cholesterol.

Abnormalities of intestinal function can alter the secretion of products that undergo enterohepatic circulation. For example, if the terminal ileum is diseased or removed, bile salt absorption is reduced. This decreases the bile salt pool (and hence bile salt secretion) and increases synthesis of bile acids by the liver. In addition, bile acids that enter the colon induce water secretion by the colonic mucosa and cause diarrhea.

■ CLINICAL TESTS

The major tests of bile secretion revolve around the measurement of serum levels of endogenous substances normally secreted in the bile, the measurement of secretion of exogenous substances injected into the blood, and the x-ray, scintigraphic, and ultrasonographic visualizations of the biliary tract.

Plasma levels of both bile salts and bile pigments are elevated in many types of hepatobiliary disease. Of these substances, bilirubin is the most commonly measured entity. Abnormalities in hepatic function can often be detected before the elevation of serum bilirubin and the development of jaundice. This is done by intravenously injecting chemicals such as sulfobromophthalein and indocyanine green. These substances normally are taken up and secreted by the same anionic transport system utilized for the hepatic secretion of bile pigments. Impairment of hepatocyte function is characterized by a slower than normal disappearance of these injected substances from the blood.

Many **gallstones** are radiopaque and can be visualized on a plain abdominal x-ray. Others, however, are radiolucent and thus not obvious. A radiopaque dye is required to facilitate visualization of these stones. The dye usually consists of iodinated anions that are taken up and secreted by the anionic transport system of the hepatocytes. The stones are then surrounded by the dye and appear as holes in the contrast medium. Radiopaque dyes are effective only if the anionic transport system of the hepatocytes is functional; therefore the tests do not work in the presence of jaundice. Scintigraphy and especially ultrasound are becoming routine for the confirmation or exclusion of gallstone disease. Ultrasonography can provide information about the thickness of the gallbladder wall, the presence of intramural gas, and even about the diameter of intrahepatic and extrahepatic bile ducts.

■ SUMMARY

1. Bile is secreted by the liver as a complex mixture of bile acids, phospholipids, cholesterol, bile pigments, electrolytes, and water.

2. Primary bile acids are synthesized from cholesterol by the hepatocytes and conjugated to taurine and glycine. Conjugated bile acids are amphipathic and, along with phospholipids and cholesterol, form mixed micelles in aqueous solution at pH values found in the intestine. Micelles take part in the digestion and absorption of dietary lipids and lipid soluble substances.

3. Hepatic bile secretion depends primarily upon the secretion of bile acids. Bile acid secretion in turn depends upon hepatocyte uptake of bile acids from the portal blood and on bile acid synthesis. Bile secretion depends to a lesser degree upon electrolyte secretion by hepatocytes and ductule cells.

4. During the fasting state, most secreted bile is stored in the gallbladder, where electrolytes and water are absorbed, thus concentrating the bile acids as an isosmotic micellar solution. Small amounts of bile empty into the duodenum during the MMC.

5. During the fed state, the gallbladder contracts, thus expelling larger quantities of bile into the duodenum. Gallbladder contraction is due mostly to the action of CCK that is released from the upper intestine in response to food products.

6. In the intestine some bile acids are deconjugated, and some primary bile acids are dehydroxylated to form secondary bile acids. These, along with the still conjugated primary bile acids, are absorbed from the intestine either passively along the length of intestine or actively, through a sodium-coupled transport process in the ileum. Once absorbed into the portal circulation, bile acids are returned to the liver, where they are actively absorbed by a sodium-coupled transport process, conjugated (if need be) and resecreted. This pattern of bile acid secretion, absorption, and resecretion is termed the enterohepatic circulation.

■ KEY WORDS AND CONCEPTS

- Bile
- Bile acids
- Micelles
- Critical micellar concentration
- Phospholipids
- Cholesterol
- Bile pigments
- Inorganic ions
- Gallbladder
- Enterohepatic circulation
- Liver
- Hepatocytes
- Bilirubin
- Hemoglobin
- Bile acid dependent secretion
- Bile acid independent secretion
- Bile duct
- Sphincter of Oddi
- Cholecystokinin
- Jaundice
- Obstruction
- Bacterial infections
- Gallstones

◼ BIBLIOGRAPHY

Hofmann AF: Biliary secretion and excretion. In Johnson LR, editor: *Physiology of the gastrointestinal tract*, vol 2, ed 3, New York, 1994, Raven Press.

Moseley RH: Bile secretion. In Yamada T, editor: *Textbook of gastroenterology*, vol 1, ed 2, Philadelphia, 1995, JB Lippincott.

Scharschmidt BF: Bilirubin metabolism, bile formation, and gallbladder and bile duct function. In Sleisenger MH, Fordtran JS, editors: *Gastrointestinal disease*, vol 2, ed 5, Philadelphia, 1993, WB Saunders.

Digestion and Absorption

Leonard R. Johnson

Motility and secretion are regulated to ensure the efficient digestion of food and absorption of nutrients across the mucosa of the gastrointestinal (GI) tract. This chapter explains how food is broken down into small absorbable molecules and how these products are transported into the blood.

■ STRUCTURAL-FUNCTIONAL ASSOCIATIONS

Food assimilation takes place primarily in the small intestine and is aided by anatomic modifications that increase the luminal surface area— Kerkring's folds, villi, and microvilli. The microvilli are prominent on the apical surface of columnar epithelial cells or enterocytes and occur to a lesser extent on goblet cells. Collectively the microvillous region comprises the **brush border.**

Several cell types make up the intestinal epithelium. Students of digestive and absorptive physiology are most familiar with **enterocytes** and **goblet cells.** Enterocytes function in digestion, absorption, and secretion. Goblet cells secrete mucus. The function of mucus is not clear but may be related to physical, chemical, and immunologic protection. Both enterocytes and goblet cells are derived from a common stem cell within the intestinal crypts. Enterocytes and goblet cells become differentiated as they move upward from the base of the crypt, and their characteristics are expressed more strongly as they migrate farther up the villus. As they reach the tip of the villus the cells are extruded and become a component of the succus entericus. In humans the time needed to replace the entire population of epithelial cells (the cell turnover time) is 3 to 6 days. Cell proliferation, differentiation, and maturation are influenced by GI hormones, growth factors, other endocrine substances, and the nature of the material in the lumen. These processes are also altered by starvation, irradiation, and loss of a portion of the bowel. The rapid proliferative rate of the intestinal mucosa makes it vulnerable to radiation and chemotherapy, procedures used to treat cancer. Despite the interplay between a basic dynamic process and the extrinsic factors that affect epithelial development, under normal conditions the mucosal appearance remains relatively constant.

■ DIGESTION

Digestion is the chemical breakdown of food by enzymes secreted by glandular cells in the mouth, chief cells in the stomach, and the exocrine cells of the pancreas, or bound to the apical membranes of enterocytes. Although some digestion of carbohydrates, proteins, and fats takes place in the stomach, the final breakdown of these substances occurs in the small intestine.

The enzymes important in digestion are summarized in Figure 11-1. **Luminal or cavital digestion** is due to enzymes secreted by the salivary glands, stomach, and pancreas. Significant chemical degradation of food is carried out, also, by hydrolytic enzymes associated with the small intestinal brush border. Hydrolysis by these enzymes is termed **contact or membrane digestion.** "Membrane" digestion is a more acceptable term, because "contact" digestion connotes activity by exogenous enzymes that become adsorbed on the epithelial surface. Membrane digestion refers to hydrolysis by enzymes synthesized by epithelial cells and inserted into the apical membrane as integral components. The half-life of membrane-bound enzymes (such as oligosaccharidases) is less than that of the epithelial cells. Thus breakdown and resynthesis occur several times during the life of a single cell.

Digestion and absorption of essentially all major dietary products take place in the small intestine. Despite the degradation of colonic contents by bacteria, physiologically important digestion does not occur in the colon. Nonetheless, absorption in this organ is impressive. A practical illustration is that some medications administered as rectal suppositories are systemically functional. During health the principal substances absorbed from the colon are water and electrolytes. However, life is possible without this organ, as evidenced by patients who thrive after colectomy.

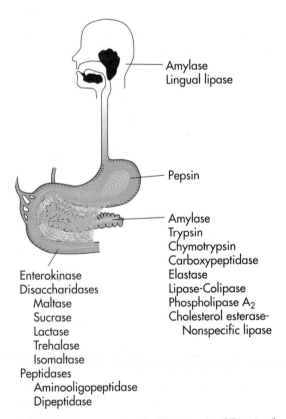

Amylase
Lingual lipase

Pepsin

Amylase
Trypsin
Chymotrypsin
Carboxypeptidase
Elastase
Lipase-Colipase
Phospholipase A_2
Cholesterol esterase-
    Nonspecific lipase

Enterokinase
Disaccharidases
    Maltase
    Sucrase
    Lactase
    Trehalase
    Isomaltase
Peptidases
    Aminooligopeptidase
    Dipeptidase

Figure 11-1 ■ Source of the principal luminal and membrane-bound digestive enzymes.

■ ABSORPTION

Although the brush border is the site of activity for a number of digestive enzymes, it is also the barrier that must be traversed by nutrients, water, and electrolytes on the way to the blood or lymph. The terms *transport* and *absorption* often are used interchangeably to mean the movement of materials from the intestinal lumen into the blood. *Secretion* implies movement in the opposite direction.

Mucosal Membrane

Conceptually the plasma membrane of the enterocyte often is considered the only factor restricting the free movement of substances from the gut lumen into the blood or lymph. However, transmural movement actually takes place over a complex pathway. This is conveyed schematically in Figure 11-2 and includes (1) an **unstirred layer of fluid,** (2) the **glycocalyx** ("fuzzy coat") covering the microvilli, (3) the cell membrane, (4) the cytoplasm of the enterocyte, (5) the basal or lateral cell membrane, (6) the intercellular space, (7) the basement membrane, and (8) the membrane of the capillary or lymph vessel.

Transport Processes

An outstanding property of the enterocyte membrane is its capacity to control the flux of solutes and fluid between the lumen and blood. This involves several mechanisms. Pinocytosis occurs at the base of microvilli and may be a major mechanism in the uptake of protein. Other uptake processes include **passive diffusion, facilitated diffusion,** and **active transport.** In the case of passive diffusion, the epithelium behaves like an inert barrier and the particles traverse this cell layer through pores in the cell membrane or through intercellular spaces. The tight junction between apposing enterocytes (Figure 11-2)

forms a mechanical seal that prevents mixing of interstitial fluid with luminal contents. This seal, however, is relatively leaky to ions and water in certain regions of the intestine, allowing some exchange between the lumen and intercellular spaces.

■ ADAPTATION OF DIGESTIVE AND ABSORPTIVE PROCESSES

Alterations in intestinal functions in response to a variety of factors are well documented. Functional adjustments that maintain homeostasis or allow an animal to cope better with its environment are termed *adaptations*. The quality and degree of adjustment are dependent upon the type of environmental stimulus encountered. Clinical situations in which the capacity to adapt is magnified are small-bowel resection and bypass. Until recently physicians knew only that a patient subjected to one of these operations underwent an initial phase of undernutrition, steat-

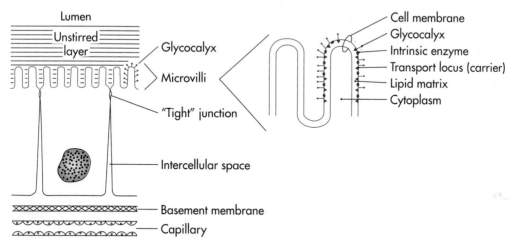

Figure 11-2 ■ Mucosal barrier. Solutes moving across the enterocyte from the intestinal lumen to the blood must traverse an unstirred layer of fluid, a glycocalyx, the apical membrane, the cytoplasm of the cell, the basolateral cell membrane, the basement membrane, and finally the wall of the capillary of the lymphatic vessel. Microvilli are morphological modifications of the cell membrane that comprise the brush border. The importance of this region in digestion and absorption of nutrients is depicted by the enlarged microvillus, which illustrates the spatial arrangement of enzymes and carrier molecules.

orrhea, and acidic diarrhea, and that these symptoms tended to be alleviated with time. Relief from the symptoms is believed to be attributable to adaptations. For example, after proximal bowel resection or bypass the remaining segment undergoes hyperplastic changes accompanied by enhancement of particular absorptive and digestive functions. Adaptation is limited in some circumstances. This point is illustrated by the fact that the absorption of vitamin B_{12} and bile salts is confined strictly to the terminal ileum. Other regions of the GI tract cannot compensate if the absorptive capacity for these compounds in the ileum is lost.

In certain genetic abnormalities, such as lactase deficiency, the capacity to adapt is lost. This condition, as well as pancreatic and intestinal diseases of varied etiology, contributes to maldigestion and malabsorption.

■ CARBOHYDRATE ASSIMILATION
Principal Dietary Forms

The average daily intake of carbohydrates, which account for approximately 50% of the calories ingested, in the United States is about 300 g. **Starch** comprises about 50% of the total, **sucrose** about 30%, **lactose** 6%, and **maltose** 1% to 2%. Trehalose, glucose, fructose, sorbitol, cellulose, hemicellulose, and pectins make up most of the remainder. Starch is a high–molecular weight compound consisting of two polysaccharides, amylose and amylopectin. Amylose is a straight-chain polymer of glucose linked by α-1,4 glycosidic bonds. The repeating disaccharide unit is maltose. **Amylopectin,** a plant starch, is the major form of carbohydrate in the diet and is similar to amylose; however, in addition to 1,4-linkages there are 1,6-linkages for every 20 to 30 glucose units. Glycogen is a high–molecular weight polysaccharide similar to amylopectin in molecular structure but having considerably more 1,6-linkages. Maltose and trehalose are dimers of glucose in 1,4- and 1,1-linkages, re-

spectively. Sucrose is a disaccharide consisting of 1 mol of glucose bound at the number 1 carbon to the number 2 carbon of fructose. Lactose is 1 mol of galactose bound at the number 1 carbon to the number 4 carbon of glucose in a β-linkage.

Digestion

Luminal digestion of starch begins in the mouth with the action of salivary α-amylase and ends in the small intestine through the action of pancreatic α-amylase. Human salivary and pancreatic amylases have optimum activities near neutral pH and are activated by Cl^-. Although salivary amylase is destroyed by acid in the stomach, some enzymatic activity occurs within the bolus of food. Most starch digestion, however, occurs in the small intestine. Hydrolysis occurs not only in the lumen but also at the surface of epithelial cells because some amylase is adsorbed to the brush border.

Amylase attacks only the interior α-1,4-bonds of amylose, yielding maltose and the trisaccharide maltotriose. Hydrolysis of amylopectin and glycogen yields similar products plus α-limit dextrins (Figure 11-3). The latter are oligosaccharides of glucose, formed because the α-1,6-linkages and the α-1,4-bonds near the 1,6-linkages are resistant to amylase. As much as one third of amylopectin cannot be hydrolyzed by amylase. The average α-limit dextrin contains 5 to 10 glucose residues and is rapidly hydrolyzed by membrane bound enzymes.

Products of amylase action on starch and other major dietary sugars are hydrolyzed by brush border carbohydrases. The process (Fig-

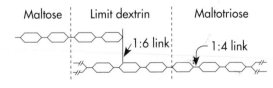

Figure 11-3 ■ Products of starch hydrolysis by α-amylase.

ure 11-4) begins with the removal of α-limit dextrins. Glucoamylase is the most active enzyme, but sucrase and isomaltase also cleave these bonds. The glucose residues are removed sequentially from the nonreducing ends until a 1-6 branch point is reached. This bond is hydrolyzed by isomaltase, which is also called α-dextrinase. Sucrase cleaves 100% of sucrose to yield glucose and fructose. All lactose is broken down into glucose and galactose by lactase. Trehalase breaks the α-1,1-bonds of trehalase into glucose. Sucrase, lactase, and trehalase break down sucrose, lactose, and trehalose, respectively.

Sucrase and isomaltase occur together as a molecular complex. The fact that congenital deficiencies of sucrase and α-dextrinase occur together reveals a close functional relationship between these two enzymes. In humans sucrase-isomaltase is a compound molecule, one unit with absolute specificity for sucrose and one for the α-1,6-linkage of an α-limit dextrin.

In general there is a large disaccharidase reserve in the small intestine, so much that the rate-limiting step in sugar assimilation is not digestion but the absorption of free hexoses following hydrolysis. Under normal circumstances the major portion of sugar assimilation is complete in the proximal jejunum. The human GI tract does not possess cellulase capable of digesting β-glucose bonds of cellulose and hemicellulose. These car-

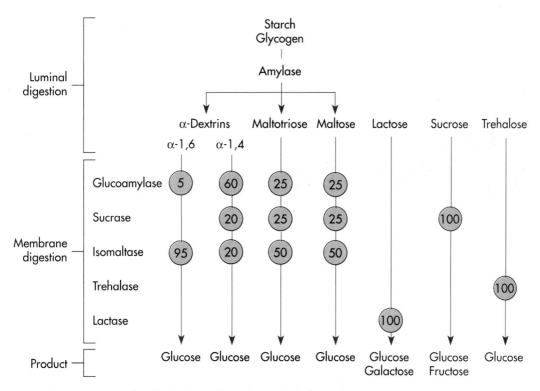

Figure 11-4 ■ **Summary of carbohydrate digestion. Circled numbers denote the approximate percent of substrate hydrolyzed by a particular brush border enzyme. The same carrier actively transports glucose and galactose into the cell, while fructose is absorbed by facilitated diffusion.**

bohydrates account for the undigestible fiber present in the diet.

Absorption of Digestion Products

For the body to utilize food-derived monosaccharides, they must be absorbed. Figure 11-5 shows how glucose absorption from the intestine occurs by passive as well as active processes. Although there are aqueous channels between enterocytes and pores in brush border membranes, dietary hexoses are too large to penetrate the membranes in any significant degree by passive diffusion. In humans the major route of entry into enterocytes is by brush border membrane carrier systems.

Fructose is transported by facilitated diffusion. In some animals it is metabolized partly to glucose, which in turn enters the circulation as it leaves the enterocytes. In humans such metabolism is minimal.

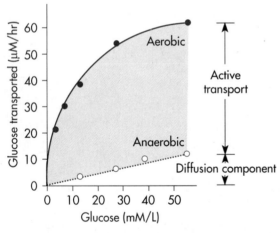

Figure 11-5 ▪ Absorption rates of glucose from a solution perfused through the intestine of a guinea pig. In the absence of oxygen the rate of mediated uptake is proportional to concentration. When oxygen is available for cellular respiration the uptake is greater, and the carrier system can be energized for active transport. (Modified from Ricklis E, Quastel JH: *Can J Biochem Physiol* 36:348-362, 1958.)

The carrier systems for fructose and glucose-galactose differ insofar as the fructose carrier cannot be energized for active transport, whereas the glucose carrier can. Glucose and galactose are absorbed by secondary active transport via a Na^+-dependent carrier system (Figure 11-6). Mutual inhibition of glucose or galactose transport by the presence of the other indicates that they are transported by a common carrier.

The glucose entry step depicted in Figure 11-6 involves a carrier that binds sodium and glucose molecules; two Na^+ for each glucose molecule are transported into the cell. The entry step is only slightly reversible because of removal of intracellular Na^+ by the pump on the basolateral membrane. Energy input (adenosine triphosphate [ATP]) drives the sodium pump and maintains a Na^+ gradient favoring glucose entry. Inhibition of the Na^+,K^+-ATPase with specific chemicals (such as ouabain) or interference in cellular energy production leads to cytosolic accumulation of Na^+ and the abolition of active sugar transport. The exit of glucose from the cytosol into the intracellular space is attributed partly to diffusion but mostly to facilitated diffusion via a Na^+-independent carrier located at the basolateral membrane.

Regulation of Absorption

The capacity of the human small intestine to absorb free sugars is enormous. It has been estimated that hexoses equivalent to 22 pounds of sucrose could be absorbed daily. There appears to be little physiologic control of sugar absorption. However, chemoreceptors and osmoreceptors in the proximal small intestine control the motility and emptying of the stomach through a negative feedback process mediated by hormones and neural reflexes. As an example, a volume of isotonic citrate solution of 750 ml placed in the human stomach passes into the small bowel in 20 minutes. The volume delivered in the same time is reduced if sucrose or glucose is added to the citrate solution. The amount delivered is related inversely to the sugar concentration.

Abnormalities in Carbohydrate Assimilation

It is obvious from the foregoing consideration that polysaccharides and oligosaccharides are absorbed not as such but as monosaccharides. Carbohydrates remaining in the intestinal lumen increase the osmotic pressure of the luminal contents because of defects in digestion and absorption. Bacterial fermentation of these carbohydrates in the lower small intestine and colon adds to this osmotic effect. The osmotic retention of water in the lumen leads to diarrhea.

Diarrhea caused by the poor assimilation of dietary carbohydrates most commonly is caused by deficiencies in carbohydrate-splitting enzymes in the intestinal brush border. **Lactase deficiency,** the most frequently observed congenital disaccharidase deficiency (which may also be acquired in later life), can exist in the absence of any other intestinal malfunction. Intolerance of sucrose and isomaltose is a rare disease found primarily in children. Intolerance of maltose has not been documented. The observation that lactase deficiency is a relatively common genetic disease, while maltase deficiency is not, may be related to the fact that only one enzyme displays significant lactase activity, whereas several dis-

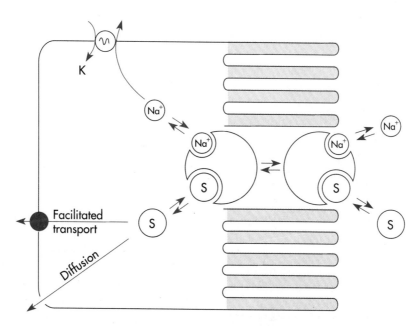

Figure 11-6 ■ Summary of a sodium-dependent carrier system for glucose-galactose. Absorption involves the rapid movement from lumen to blood by an entry step and exit step mediated by two separate carrier molecules with specificity for hexose. The system is energized by an ATP-dependent Na^+ pump that maintains sodium gradient favoring the entry of Na^+ into the cell, with the concomitant co-transport of substrate *(S)*. When Na^+ is pumped from the cell, more Na^+ and glucose are transported into the cell from the lumen. The transport capacity of the carrier involved in glucose exit appears to equal that involved in glucose entry because glucose does not accumulate within the cells to a large degree.

play activity against maltose (Figure 11-4). Thus maltose intolerance would require the simultaneous absence of all enzymes possessing maltase activity. Maldigestion of starch in humans in nonexistent, because pancreatic amylase is secreted in tremendous excess.

Intolerance to glucose and galactose has been documented in rare instances. In these cases the patients thrive and show no symptoms when fed fructose. The explanation for this is found in the specificity of sugar absorption. Glucose and chemically related sugars are absorbed by a Na^+-dependent secondary active transport process, whereas fructose is absorbed by Na^+-independent facilitated diffusion. In these patients the carrier for glucose is absent.

Besides defects in carbohydrate assimilation caused by the congenital or acquired enzyme deficiencies, assimilation of dietary sugars may be impaired by diseases of the GI tract. Celiac disease, certain bacterial infections, and some protozoan and helminth infections are associated with inflammation and structural derangements in the small bowel mucosa. These conditions often are attended by brush border enzyme deficiencies and hexose malabsorption (Figure 11-7). It is not uncommon to find lactase deficiency as a long-term consequence of intestinal disease, because this enzyme is present in the intestine at low levels compared with maltase and sucrase.

Symptoms of osmotic diarrhea include cramps and abdominal distention. An oral tolerance test can be used to diagnose disaccharidase deficiency if this is a suspected cause. After an overnight fast, adult patients are fed 50 g of lactose in a 10% aqueous solution (children are usually fed 2 g/kg body weight). Blood samples are taken for glucose analysis before and at 5, 10, 15, 30, 45, and 60 minutes after lactose administration. An increase in blood glucose of at least 25 mg/dl over fasted levels indicates normal hydrolysis of lactose and normal absorption of the glu-

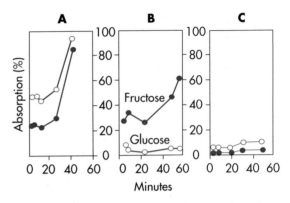

Figure 11-7 ■ *Relative rates of absorption of fructose and glucose in an equimolar mixture studied by an intubation technique in A, a control subject; B, a patient with glucose malabsorption; and C, a patient with celiac disease.* (From Dahlquist A: In Sipple HL, McNutt KW, editor: *Sugars in nutrition,* New York, 1974, Academic Press.)

cose product. A flat lactose tolerance curve or failure to observe a rise in blood glucose over 25 mg/dl following lactose ingestion indicates low lactase activity. A value between 20 and 25 mg/dl is questionable. In this case the test may be repeated; or, if laboratory facilities permit, intestinal biopsy specimens can be collected and examined for enzyme activity. In dealing with biopsy specimens, enzyme activity usually is expressed as units per gram of tissue protein. Tolerance tests for disaccharides other than lactose are seldom performed, but a similar procedure would suffice. Glucose or galactose tolerance tests should be performed to exclude monosaccharide malabsorption as the cause of a flat lactose tolerance curve.

■ PROTEIN ASSIMILATION
Digestion

Protein digestion begins in the stomach with the action of pepsin. The enzyme precursor, pepsinogen, is secreted by chief cells in response to a meal and low gastric pH. Acid in the stomach is responsible for activating pepsinogen to pepsin.

Three pepsin isozymes have been recognized. All have a pH optimum of 1 to 3 and are denatured above pH 5. Pepsin is an endopeptidase with specificity for peptide bonds involving aromatic L-amino acids.

Pepsin activity terminates when the gastric contents mix with alkaline pancreatic juice in the small bowel. Food in the intestine stimulates the release of secretin and cholecystokinin (CCK), which in turn causes the pancreas to secrete bicarbonate and enzymes into the intestinal lumen.

There are two general classes of pancreatic proteases, **endopeptidases** and **exopeptidases.** The basis of classification and the particular characteristics of specific enzymes belonging to each class are given in Table 11-1.

Pancreatic proteases are secreted into the duodenum as inactive precursors. **Trypsinogen,** which lacks proteolytic activity, is activated by **enterokinase,** an enzyme located on the brush border of duodenal enterocytes. The exact chemical composition of enterokinase is not known; however, the fact that the molecule is 41% carbohydrate probably prevents its rapid digestion by proteolytic enzymes. The activity of enterokinase is stimulated by trypsinogen, and it is released from the brush border membrane by bile salts. Enterokinase activates trypsinogen by releasing a hexapeptide from the N-terminal end of the precursor molecule (Figure 11-8). Active trypsin, once formed, acts autocatalytically in the manner of enterokinase to activate the bulk of trypsinogen. Trypsin also activates other peptidase precursors from the pancreas (Figure 11-8). **Chymotrypsinogen** is activated by cleavage of the peptide bond between arginine and isoleucine, which are the fifteenth and sixteenth amino acid residues at the N-terminus. Although structural rearrangement occurs, no peptide fragment is released because of a disulfide bond between the cysteine residues at positions 1 and 122 in the protein chain. This configuration is the active form of chymotrypsinogen. Cleavage at other points in the chymotrypsinogen molecule produces other molecular species of chymotrypsin having relatively little physiologic importance. The exact mechanism for activation of **proelastase** is not known and activation of **procarboxypeptidases A and B** is relatively

---

T A B L E   1 1 - 1

Principal pancreatic proteases

Enzyme	Primary action
Endopeptidases	Hydrolyze interior peptide bonds of polypeptides and proteins
Trypsin	Attacks peptide bonds involving basic amino acids; yields products with basic amino acids at C-terminal end
Chymotrypsin	Attacks peptide bonds involving aromatic amino acids, leucine, glutamine, and methionine; yields peptide products with these amino acids at C-terminal end
Elastase	Attacks peptide bonds involving neutral aliphatic amino acids; yields products with neutral amino acids at C-terminal end
Exopeptidases	Hydrolyze external peptide bonds of polypeptides and protein
Carboxypeptidase A	Attacks peptides with aromatic and neutral aliphatic amino acids at C-terminal end
Carboxypeptidase B	Attacks peptides with basic amino acids at C-terminal end

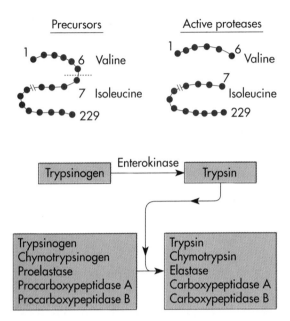

Figure 11-8 ▪ Activation of pancreatic proteolytic enzymes.

complicated, involving proteolysis of at least two proenzymes.

Once in the small intestine, pancreatic enzymes undergo rapid inactivation because of autodigestion. Trypsin is the enzyme primarily responsible for inactivation.

Absorption of Digestion Products

Membrane digestion and absorption are closely related phenomena in protein assimilation, and physiologists have been occupied by two fundamental questions concerning them: (1) In what form do products of proteolysis cross the brush border membrane of the epithelial cell? (2) In what form do these products lease the cell to enter the blood?

L-Isomers of some amino acids are absorbed by carrier-mediated mechanisms in much the same manner as glucose is absorbed. As with glucose the cell entry process requires Na$^+$ as part of a ternary complex (Figure 11-6), and uphill

transfer occurs by secondary active transport. Other amino acids and some of those absorbed by active transport can also be absorbed by facilitated diffusion processes that do not require Na$^+$ (Table 11-2).

Certain L-amino acids compete with one another for uptake by intestinal cells. Studies of competition have led to the recognition of several different carrier systems for amino acid absorption (Table 11-2). There is little doubt that the absorption of free amino acids by gut mucosa is physiologically important. However, amino acids appear in portal blood faster and reach a higher level when peptides from an acid hydrolysate of protein contact the gut mucosa than when there is an equimolar solution of free amino acid (Figure 11-9). Also, greater amounts of total nitrogen are absorbed from a solution of trypsin hydrolysate of proteins than from an equivalent solution of amino acids in free form. Competition for transport between two chemically related amino acids is not observed when the same two acids are absorbed after ingestion of their dipeptides and tripeptides. In addition, the site in the intestine for the maximum absorption of amino acids in small peptide form is different from that for the absorption of free amino acid. The current explanation of these findings is that a separate carrier system for small peptides is involved in absorption. For example, free glycine absorption requires an amino acid carrier system. If saturation of the system occurs under physiologic conditions, the maximum rate of uptake becomes limiting. If, however, a second carrier for dipeptides or tripeptides of glycine is present, the amino acids can enter the cell in small-peptide form. Thus two separate systems for glycine entry exist and work in a parallel manner.

The prevailing concepts regarding protein assimilation are illustrated in Figure 11-10. Luminal digestion of a protein meal produces approximately 40% free amino acids and 60% small pep-

Carrier systems for the transport of amino acids

Transport system	Substrates	Dependence on Na$^+$ gradient
Brush Border Membrane		
Neutral	All neutral aromatic and aliphatic AA	Yes
PHE	Phenylalanine and methionine	Yes
Acidic	Glutamate, aspartate	Yes
Imino	Proline, hydroxyproline	Yes
y$^+$	Basic AA	No
L	Neutral AA with hydrophobic side chains	No
Basolateral Membrane		
A	Small neutral AA	Yes
ASC	Three and four carbon neutral AA	Yes
L	Neutral AA with hydrophobic side chains	No
y$^+$	Basic AA	No

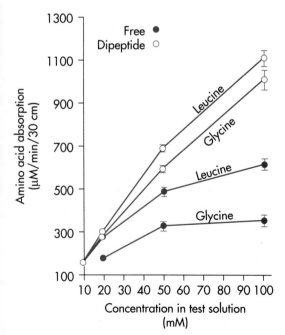

Figure 11-9 ■ **Jejunal rates of glycine and leucine absorption (mean ± SEM, five subjects) from perfusion of test solutions containing either L-glycyl-L-leucine or an equimolar mixture of free L-glycine and free L-leucine.** (From Adibi SA: *J Clin Invest* 50:2266-2275, 1971.)

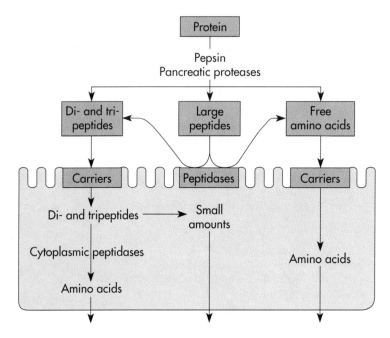

Figure 11-10 ■ **Summary of the digestion and absorption of protein. Luminal digestion yields 40% free amino acids and 60% peptides consisting primarily of 2 to 6 amino acid residues.**

tides. As with the free acids, dipeptides and tripeptides resulting from digestion can be absorbed intact by carrier-mediated processes. However, tetra-, penta-, and hexapeptides are poorly absorbed; instead they are hydrolyzed by brush border peptidases to free amino acids or smaller absorbable peptides. Small peptides are probably absorbed by a single carrier with broad specificity. This is a secondary active transport process dependent on the Na^+ gradient.

Peptides that enter enterocytes are hydrolyzed by cytoplasmic peptidases to amino acids. These, in turn, diffuse or are moved by carrier-mediated processes from the intracellular compartment, across the basolateral membrane, into the blood. As was the case with the apical membrane, a number of different carriers exist in the basolateral membrane (Table 11-2). Some of these are also Na^+ dependent. A small percentage of peptides enter the blood intact, which

may explain why certain biologically active peptides exert their effects when given orally.

Abnormalities in Protein Assimilation

Pancreatic insufficiency caused by various diseases, including cystic fibrosis and hereditary pancreatitis, may be associated with a decrease or absence of trypsin and may lead to poor digestion of protein. Cases of primary proteinase deficiency caused by congenital trypsinogen deficiency have been reported. In those patients, chymotrypsin and carboxypeptidase activities are lacking also, because trypsin cannot be formed to activate the precursors of these pancreatic proteases.

Intestinal malabsorption of amino acids occurs in various hereditary diseases. Knowledge of intestinal transport abnormalities of this type is important, not only for understanding the pathogenesis of certain diseases but also for providing important information regarding the physiologic process involved in intestinal transport.

Cystinuria is a disease characterized partly by defective transport of cystine in the proximal renal tubule and the small bowel (Figure 11-11). Although the intestinal malabsorptive condition is of little or no consequence in the disability produced by cystinuria, the fact that it is limited to the basic amino acids is supportive evidence that specific carrier systems exist for the intestinal uptake of amino acids.

Hartnup disease is a hereditary condition in which the active transport of several neutral amino acids is deficient in both the renal tubules and the small intestine. The intestinal defect contributes to the pathogenesis of this disorder. An interesting finding is that, although neutral amino acids are not absorbed, they readily appear in the blood when their dipeptides are fed to patients. This is compelling evidence that absorption of the dipeptides of certain amino acids is by a completely separate process from the one involved in the transport of free amino acids.

■ LIPID ASSIMILATION

Dietary lipids are complex organic compounds and include such substances as phospholipids, sterols, hydrocarbons, and waxes that comprise cell walls or membranes of plants and/or animals. Other lipids or related dietary constituents are fat droplets (triglycerides) and fat-soluble vitamins (A, D, E, K). The principles of lipid assimilation are dealt with through a consideration of **triglycerides, phospholipids,** and **sterols.** The propensity of lipids to form ester linkages and the insolubility of lipids in water are important properties to keep in mind in relation to digestion and absorption.

Unlike carbohydrates and proteins, lipids enter epithelial cells by a sequence of chemical and physical events that render water-insoluble molecules capable of being absorbed by passive diffusion. The process depends upon four major

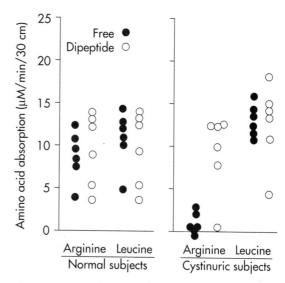

Figure 11-11 ■ Jejunal absorption of free arginine and leucine during perfusion of solutions containing L-arginine (1 mM) and L-leucine (1 mM) or L-arginyl-L-leucine (1 mM). Results are from studies carried out in six normal subjects and six cystinuric patients. (From Silk DBA, Dawson AM: In Crane RK, Guyton AC, editors: *International review of physiology. III, Gastrointestinal physiology,* Baltimore, 1979, University Park Press.)

events: (1) secretion of bile and various lipases, (2) emulsification, (3) enzymatic hydrolysis of ester linkages, and (4) the solubilization of lipolytic products within bile salt micelles.

Digestion

Fat assimilation begins in the stomach, where food (partially digested by pepsin) is churned into a coarse mixture and released in small portions into the duodenum. Except for short-chain fatty acids, there is no absorption of fat from the stomach. There is a process, controlled through the action of CCK, that slows gastric motility and emptying when fat is in the small intestine. CCK also stimulates the pancreas to secrete lipase and causes contraction of the gallbladder. One function of bile salts released into the duodenum is to perpetuate the **emulsification** of fat droplets by decreasing the surface tension at the oil-water interface. An emulsification is a suspension of fat droplets held apart by lecithin, bile salts, fatty acids, and other emulsifying agents. The emulsified fat droplets are approximately 1 μm in diameter. The emulsification process is important to increasing the surface area of lipids in preparation for their enzymatic hydrolysis.

Enzymes from four sources are involved in the digestion of dietary lipids. These include food-bearing lipases, lingual lipase, gastric lipase and pancreatic lipases.

Enzymes that digest dietary lipids can be found in food per se (e.g., acid lipases and phospholipases). These enzymes may function in autodigestion, a process aided by the acid environment of the stomach. Human milk contains a lipase similar in chemical properties to bile salt–stimulated lipase secreted by the pancreas. Known as **carboxylic ester hydrolase** (CEH), it is active against cholesterol and vitamin A esters. Milk lipase and CEH also hydrolyze glycerol esters of long-chain fatty acids at the physiologic pH of the small bowel. A feature that distinguishes these esterases from well-known pancreatic lipase is that the latter has pronounced specificity for the 1 and 3 ester bonds of triglycerides, whereas milk lipase and CEH show no positional specificity. Despite the lack of a clear functional role, it is presumed that milk lipase working in conjunction with CEH is important to the utilization of milk lipids in newborn infants, who have a low intestinal bile salt concentration and absorb glycerol and free fatty acids better than monoglycerides. This presumption is compatible with knowledge that milk lipase is stable between pH 3.5 and 9 and is broken down only slowly by pepsin. Thus most of the enzyme would pass through the infant's stomach without denaturation. The fact that it requires bile salts for activation suggests that it is not functional until it reaches the small intestine.

Lipolytic activity in the human stomach is due primarily to **gastric lipase** secreted by cells of the fundus. Lingual lipase is much less important in the human. Both of these enzymes have acidic pH optima, ranging from 3 to 6. Gastric lipase acts primarily at the outer ester linkages, producing fatty acids and diglycerides. Pancreatic lipase normally is produced in great excess, and the absence of gastric lipase would not alter fat digestion. However, the contribution of gastric lipase can be significant in newborns and patients with pancreatic lipase deficiency or inactivation, such as might occur in Zollinger-Ellison syndrome because of the acid environment of the duodenum.

Pancreatic lipase-colipase, phospholipase A_2, and cholesterol esterase (nonspecific lipase) all function within the intestinal lumen.

Pancreatic lipase, or glycerol-ester lipase, is secreted in an active form rather than as a precursor enzyme. It displays optimum activity at pH 8 and remains active down to pH 3.0. A more acidic pH destroys the enzyme. Although bile salts inhibit its enzymatic activity, this is prevented under physiologic circumstances by the combination of lipase with **colipase.** Colipase, a polypeptide (102 to 107 amino acids) secreted by the pancreas along with lipase is a 1:1 ratio, is secreted as procolipase that is activated when hydrolyzed by trypsin to a peptide containing 96 amino acids. Whereas lipase-colipase complexes are scarce within the duodenum during fasting, the presence of fat stimulates the secretion of these components in large quantities. The inactivation of lipase by bile salts and the prevention or reversal of inactivation by colipase due, respectively, to the capacity of bile salts to displace lipase at the fat droplet–water interface, where it must exert its action, and to the obverse capacity of colipase to replace the bile salts at this interface. Once colipase attaches to the fat droplet, lipase will bind to a specific site on the colipase molecule in a 1:1 ratio and consequently carry out its catalytic function, breaking down triglycerides. Colipase also has the capacity to bind to a bile salt micelle. Therefore the products of fat hydrolysis might be transferred directly to a micelle.

Lipase is secreted in large excess and rapidly hydrolyzes triglycerides. The enzyme shows positional specificity. It cleaves the 1 and 3 ester linkages, yielding free fatty acids and 2-monoglycerides. Only small amounts of free glycerol (Figure 11-12) are produced, reflecting the lack of action against the 2 ester linkages.

Phospholipase A₂ is secreted as a proenzyme and is activated by trypsin much in the same fashion as trypsinogen is converted to active form (i.e., through cleavage of several amino acids from the N-terminus). Bile salts and phospholipids form mixed micelles that become substrates for phospholipase A₂. The enzyme has an absolute requirement for bile salts in hydrolyzing dietary phospholipids at the 2 position and producing lysophospholipid and free fatty acids.

Human pancreatic **cholesterol esterase** hydrolyzes not only cholesterol esters but also the esters of vitamins A, D, and E, as well as those of glycerides. In contrast to pancreatic lipase,

cholesterol esterase hydrolyzes all three ester linkages of triglycerides. This capacity accounts for its name, **nonspecific esterase.** Cholesterol esterase is active against substrates that have been incorporated into bile salt micelles. Activity apparently is dependent on the presence of specific bile salts. The enzyme in humans attacks cholesterol ester in the presence of taurocholate and taurochenodeoxycholate. Esterases from other species may have different bile salt requirements.

Cholesterol esterase is present also in small intestinal epithelial cells. Because the enzyme can catalyze the synthesis of cholesterol esters as well as break them down, it is postulated to function in the formation of chylomicrons.

Absorption of Lipolytic Products

In addition to the function just mentioned, bile salts perform an important function in the actual absorption of lipolytic products. Sodium glycocholic and taurocholic acids, which are major bile salts, have both hydrophobic and hydrophilic portions. When their concentration in the intestine is raised to a critical level, bile salt monomers form water-soluble aggregates called

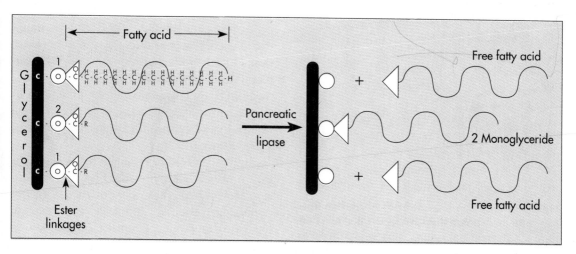

Figure 11-12 ■ Positional specificity of pancreatic lipase.

micelles. The concentration of bile salt at which molecular aggregation occurs is referred to as the **critical micellar concentration.** Conjugated bile salts have a lower critical micellar concentration than do unconjugated ones. Whereas emulsion particles are 2,000 to 50,000 Å in diameter, micelles are about 30 to 100 Å in diameter with a hydrophilic outer surface and a hydrophobic center. The water-insoluble monoglycerides from lipolysis are solubilized within the hydrophobic center of the micelle (Figure 11-13). In turn, fatty acids, lysophospholipids, cholesterol, and fat-soluble vitamins may be solubilized. A mixed micellar solution is water-clear. Micellar solubilization is important because it enhances the diffusion of poorly soluble dietary lipids through the unstirred aqueous layer overlying the enterocytes.

Two forms of evidence support the participation of micelles in the assimilation of fatty substances. First, mixed micelles (bile salts plus lipids) are found in the intestine. Second, long-chain fatty acids and monoglycerides are ab-

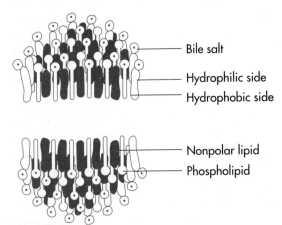

Figure 11-13 ■ Solubilization of nonpolar lipid by a bile acid–polar lipid micelle. (Modified from Hoffman AF, French A, Littman A: *Syllabus. Digestion and absorption,* Chicago, 1975, American Medical Association.)

Bile salt
Hydrophilic side
Hydrophobic side

Nonpolar lipid
Phospholipid

sorbed more rapidly from micellar solution than from emulsions.

One possible mechanism of lipid uptake by enterocytes is the absorption of the entire mixed micelle. This proposed mechanism is not accepted, however, because various lipolytic products are absorbed at different rates. Also, because bile salts are absorbed in the ileum, and lipid absorption usually is completed in the midjejunum, it is unlikely that the whole micelle enters the intestinal epithelium. Once absorption takes place, bile salts are transported back to the liver for resecretion. The process of bile secretion, absorption, and return to the liver is referred to as the **enterohepatic circulation.**

The importance of micellar solubilization lies in the ability of micelles to diffuse across the unstirred water layer and present large amounts of fatty acids and monoglycerides to the apical membrane of the enterocyte. The brush border membrane is separated from the bulk solution in the intestinal lumen by the unstirred water layer. Single fatty acid and monoglyceride molecules, being poorly soluble in water, move slowly through this barrier. Since uptake depends on the number of molecules in contact with the enterocyte membrane, their absorption will be diffusion-limited. In contrast, micelles are water soluble, diffuse readily through the unstirred layer, and increase the concentration of fatty acids and monoglycerides at the membrane by 100- to 1000-fold. Short- and medium-chain fatty acids are not dependent on micelles for uptake because of their higher solubility in and diffusion through the unstirred aqueous layer.

Until recently it was thought that all fat digestion products were absorbed by simple diffusion. However, there is now evidence of carrier-dependent processes. Some products such as linoleate show saturable uptake. Uptake in some cases exhibits a specificity that cannot be part of simple diffusion.

Intracellular Events

Monoglycerides and free fatty acids absorbed by enterocytes are resynthesized into triglycerides by two different pathways: the major one, monoglyceride acylation; and the minor one, phosphatidic acid (Figure 11-14).

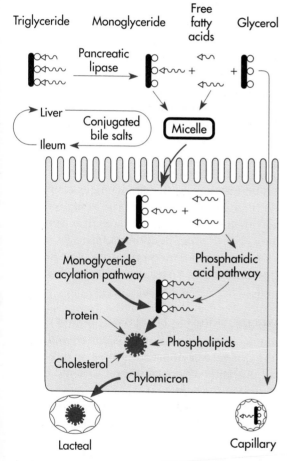

Figure 11-14 ■ **Summary of the digestion and absorption of triglyceride. Monoglycerides and long-chain fatty acids enter the cells after first being incorporated into micelles. Glycerol and short-chain and medium-chain acids, because of their solubility in the aqueous unstirred layer, enter without micelle solubilization.**

Monoglyceride Acylation Pathway The monoglyceride acylation pathway involves the synthesis of triglycerides from 2-monoglycerides and coenzyme A (CoA)–activated fatty acids. Acyl-CoA synthetase is the enzyme that acylates fatty acids. The enzymes monoglyceride and diglyceride acyltransferases are responsible for catalyzing the formation of diglycerides and triglycerides, respectively. The enzymes involved in this pathway are associated with the smooth endoplasmic reticulum.

An interesting aspect of intracellular triglyceride synthesis is that certain fatty acids are used in preference to others. This occurs despite similar rates of absorption by enterocytes and similar rates of enzymatic CoA activation and glyceride esterification. These observations have been explained by the presence of intracellular **fatty acid–binding proteins** (FABPs), which have affinities for fatty acids of different chain lengths and varying degrees of saturation. Such proteins exert their influence after absorption occurs and before esterification takes place.

A current theory on how FABPs operate presumes that absorbed fatty acids bind strongly to the apical membrane of enterocytes. Solubilization is brought about when the fatty acids bind specifically with receptors on FABPs. This facilitates the transfer of the free fatty acids from the apical membrane to the smooth endoplasmic reticulum, where esterification into diglycerides and triglycerides takes place. This process is particularly effective in the intracellular transfer of long-chain fatty acids. Short- and medium-chain fatty acids, which show less affinity for the cell membrane, are water soluble, and are not bound by specific proteins. Instead they leave the cell in free form and enter the blood directly rather than as reesterified triglyceride in chylomicrons.

Phosphatidic Acid Pathway Triglycerides also can be synthesized from CoA fatty acids and α-glycerophosphate. The latter is formed from phosphorylated glycerol or from the reduction of dihydroxyacetone phosphate derived from glycolysis. One mole of α-glycerophosphate acylated with 2 mol of CoA–fatty acids yields phosphatidic acid, which is dephosphorylated to form diglyceride, which, in turn, is acylated to form triglyceride. This minor pathway for triglyceride synthesis in the intestine is termed the *phosphatidic acid pathway.*

Phosphatidic acid may be important also in the synthesis of phospholipids such as phosphatidyl choline, ethanolamine, and serine. Alternatively, phospholipids can be derived from acylation of absorbed lysophospholipids by appropriate acyltransferases. The acylation of lysophosphatidyl choline forms phosphatidyl choline, which, along with absorbed phosphatidyl choline, is utilized in the formation of chylomicrons.

Dietary cholesterol is absorbed in free form. However, a major fraction leaves the epithelial cells in chylomicrons as esters of fatty acids. This is indicative of the highly active intracellular reesterification process. The ratio of free to esterified cholesterol in intestinal lymph is influenced by the amount of cholesterol in the diet (low dietary cholesterol favors the cellular exit of greater amounts of free sterol in chylomicrons). In humans the rate of cholesterol absorption decreases as the dietary content increases.

Chylomicrons are lipoprotein particles about 750 to 5000 Å in diameter that are synthesized within enterocytes and exist in the form of an emulsion. Although their chemical composition may vary slightly depending on size, chylomicrons are approximately 80% to 90% triglycerides, 8% to 9% phospholipids, 2% cholesterol, 2% protein, and traces of carbohydrate. It is not evident how triglycerides and esterified cholesterol and fat-soluble vitamins (which form the core) become coated with **apoprotein,** phospholipid, and free cholesterol (which make up the surface of the chylomicron). Synthesis of both triglyceride and apoprotein occurs in the endoplasmic reticulum, where they form complexes along with phospholipids. This complex, in turn, is transported to the Golgi apparatus, where the protein is glycosylated. The newly formed chylomicrons are secreted by exocytosis into the interstitial space, traverse the basement membrane, and enter the gaps between the endothelial cells comprising the lacteals. Chylomicrons are too large to enter the pores of blood capillaries.

It is evident that apoprotein synthesis by epithelial cells and its incorporation into chylomicrons are essential for fat absorption. Inhibition of protein synthesis causes large amounts of triglyceride to accumulate intracellularly. Several apoproteins (termed A, B, C, and E) have been identified in intestinal lymph. Apoprotein B is similar immunologically to plasma very-low-density lipoprotein (VLDL) and low-density lipoprotein (LDL) but chemically and physically shows some uniqueness. It has been suggested that VLDL and LDL in intestinal plasma may represent chylomicrons of varying densities. Generally, however, the role of apoproteins in fat absorption and metabolism is only vaguely understood and remains a current area of active investigation.

Abnormalities in Lipid Assimilation

Impaired lipid assimilation is considered under the general title of malabsorption. In most cases all nutrients are malabsorbed to some extent. However, the definition of the clinical entity is in terms of fat malabsorption because, unlike carbohydrates and proteins, fat not absorbed in the small intestine passes through the colon and appears in the feces in a measurable form.

Excessive fat in the stool can be established by extracting fecal samples with organic solvents and determining the total fatty acids present, excluding volatile short-chain acids. Less than 7 g of fecal fatty acid per day is normal. Values above this level suggest malabsorption.

A convenient way to consider fat malabsorption is to take the various steps in assimilation and consider possible derangements. For each derangement there is at least one possible disease:

- Disorders of gastric mixing and intestinal motility do not have any clearcut disease associated with them, although malabsorption may follow the rapid gastric emptying the accompanies partial gastrectomy. Also, rapid intestinal transit has been suggested as the basis for diarrhea in hyperthyroidism.

- Luminal digestion of triglycerides may be deranged by defects in pancreatic enzyme secretion or action. A quantitative defect would be caused by impaired enzyme synthesis and secretion, as occurs with cystic fibrosis (a congenital disease of exocrine glands) or chronic pancreatitis. It should be noted that normal digestion can proceed with as little as 10% to 15% of normal enzyme secretion. A qualitative defect would occur if the conditions for enzyme action were not optimal (as in gastric acid hypersecretion [Zollinger-Ellison syndrome], when the pH of the duodenal contents is lowered and lipase cannot function or may even be denatured).

- Transport from the lumen is a special step in fat absorption and is dependent on a suitable bile acid concentration, which may be low because of a quantitative bile acid deficiency that occurs with an interrupted enterohepatic circulation (e.g., ileal resection or dysfunction, or biliary obstruction). There may be a qualitative deficit of the bile acids in a condition known as the *bacterial overgrowth syndrome* (in which stasis in the upper intestine leads to bacterial overgrowth, with deconjugation of bile acids by the bacteria). Free bile acids are absorbed passively in the jejunum because they are largely un-ionized at the duodenal pH. Bile acids need to be ionized to form micelles.

Therefore the un-ionized state leads to impairment of fat absorption as well as impaired absorption of cholesterol and fat-soluble vitamins.

- Mucosal cell transport is, of course, necessary for all nutrients; but it is of particular importance in fat absorption, because the absorbed fatty acids or monoglycerides must be reconstituted to triglycerides and then formed into chylomicrons. No disease has been associated with triglyceride synthesis; however, there is a disease of inadequate chylomicron formation, abetalipoproteinemia.

- Lymphatic transport is necessary for the absorption of fat that has been reconstituted to chylomicrons. This step is defective in two rare diseases, congenital lymphagiectasis and Whipple's disease.

Thus by considering the steps in fat absorption it is possible to predict the diseases that can lead to malabsorption. Steatorrhea, which attends malabsorption, can be alleviated to a large degree by diets containing triglycerides of medium-rather than long-chain fatty acids. The explanation for this is that glycerol esters of medium-chain fatty acids are hydrolyzed faster than are ester linkages involving long-chain fatty acids. Medium-chain fatty acids are water soluble and can be absorbed from aqueous solution. Also they are transported directly into portal blood without involvement of chylomicrons.

■ VITAMINS

Vitamins are organic compounds that cannot be manufactured by the body but are vital for metabolism. They are considered in this instance, not on the basis of any physiologic function, but rather on the basis of whether they are water soluble or fat soluble (Table 11-3). This feature is emphasized because their solubility dictates the general mechanism by which vitamins are absorbed.

TABLE 11-3

Solubility of vitamins

Vitamin	Fat soluble	Water soluble
A	+	
B$_1$ (thiamine)		+
B$_2$ (riboflavin)		+
Niacin		+
C (ascorbic acid)		+
D	+	
E	+	
K	+	
Folic acid		+
B$_6$ (pyridoxine, pyridoxal, pyridoxamine)		+
B$_{12}$		+
Pantothenic acid		+
Biotin		+

Water-soluble vitamins are represented by an array of compounds. The principles that apply to the absorption of hexoses and amino acids apply to the absorption of vitamins as well. Strongly ionized or high–molecular weight compounds are absorbed poorly compared with nonionized, low–molecular weight substances.

Relatively little information exists regarding the processes involved in the intestinal uptake of vitamins. Most evidence suggests that passive diffusion is the predominant mechanism. Exceptions exist for thiamine, vitamin C, folic acid, and vitamin B$_{12}$, for which special transport mechanisms have been reported.

As low luminal concentrations, thiamine (vitamin B$_1$) can be absorbed in the jejunum of some species, including humans, by a Na$^+$-dependent, active process, whereas at high concentrations passive diffusion predominates. The presence of a carrier-mediated transport system is suggested by the fact that metabolic inhibitors, thiamine analogues, and the absence of sodium all depress thiamine uptake by enterocytes. Riboflavin (vitamin B$_2$) is absorbed in the proximal small bowel by facilitated transport. Pyridoxine (vitamin B$_6$) is absorbed by simple diffusion.

Vitamin C is required in only a few species, including humans. Humans are capable of absorbing it from the intestine by passive processes and also by active transport (an energy-dependent process, requiring Na$^+$). In rats and hamsters, species that do not require ascorbic acid, uptake of the vitamin occurs only by passive mechanisms.

Folic acid has been reported to be transported actively in the duodenum and jejunum of humans and from the entire small intestine of some rodents. A mediated process might be predicted from two facts: folic acid is a strongly electronegative compound (with a molecular weight of 441), and uncouplers of respiration (hence, energy production) interfere with its absorption.

Vitamin B$_{12}$ (cobalamin) absorption requires intrinsic factor, a glycoprotein secreted by the parietal cell of the gastric mucosa. Binding of intrinsic factor to dietary vitamin B$_{12}$ is necessary for attachment to specific receptors located in the brush border of the ileum. Initially cobalamin is released from foods by the action of pepsin. Because of a higher affinity for R proteins (glycoproteins), which are secreted in gastric juice along with intrinsic factor, the vitamin and R proteins form a complex. When the R protein becomes digested in the duodenum, the vitamin then forms a complex with intrinsic factor that is resistant to digestion. The presence of Ca^{++} or Mg^{++} and an alkaline pH are necessary for optimal attachment of the intrinsic factor-B$_{12}$ complex to the receptor, a process that does not require energy. The actual uptake of B$_{12}$ is presumed to be by pinocytosis; however, this point is not clear. Any disease condition that interferes with the production or secretion of intrinsic factor or with the attachment of the intrinsic factor-B$_{12}$

complex to its receptor in the ileum leads to malabsorption of vitamin B_{12}.

The fat-soluble vitamins (A, D, E, and K) depend upon solubilization within bile salt micelles for intestinal absorption. Vitamin A, or retinol, is ingested as β-carotene and absorbed as such. Once in the enterocyte, β-carotene is cleaved intracellularly into two retinol molecules. Esters of dietary vitamin D and E, as noted earlier in this chapter, are digested by cholesterol ester hydrolase before their solubilization in micelles. Dietary vitamin K (K_1) is absorbed in the intestine by an active transport system, while bacterially derived K_2 is taken up passively from the lumen. Except for retinol, which is reesterified, the fat soluble vitamins appear in exocytosed chylomicrons biochemically unaltered by metabolic processes within the enterocyte. The chylomicrons are then extruded into the lymphatics and transported via the thoracic duct into the blood.

■ SUMMARY

1. Digestion is the chemical breakdown of food by enzymes secreted into the lumen of the gut and those associated with the brush border of enterocytes.
2. All physiologically significant absorption of nutrients occurs in the small intestine, the mucosal surface of which is greatly increased providing a large area for uptake.
3. The major luminal breakdown of carbohydrates is catalyzed by amylase. Breakdown of remaining glucose polymers and other disaccharides is carried out by specific enzymes in the brush border membrane. Glucose and galactose share a Na^+-dependent, secondary active-transport mechanism for absorption.
4. The major enzymes involved in the luminal digestion of protein are secreted in inactive forms by the pancreas and then activated by trypsin following its own activation by enterokinase.
5. Di- and tripeptides and amino acids are absorbed across the brush border membrane by a variety of transport processes. Larger peptides are broken down into these absorbable forms by peptidases associated with the brush border. Absorbed small peptides are hydrolyzed to amino acids within the cytoplasm, and almost all absorbed protein leaves the enterocyte in the form of amino acids.
6. Fat droplets are suspended in an emulsification by the action of lecithin, bile salts, peptides, and other such agents. Colipase displaces a bile salt molecule from the fat-water interface, allowing pancreatic lipase to digest the triglycerides. Pancreatic lipase is essential to fat digestion and produces 2-monoglycerides and free fatty acids.
7. The breakdown products of fat digestion are solubilized in micelles by bile salts and other amphipathic molecules. Micelles diffuse through the unstirred layer, and fat digestion products are absorbed from the micelles at the enterocyte brush border membrane.
8. Within the enterocyte, triglycerides and phospholipids are resynthesized and packaged into chylomicrons that contain apoprotein on their surface. Chylomicrons are exocytosed into the intercellular space. Too large to enter capillaries, the chylomicrons enter lacteals and eventually reach the blood via the thoracic lymph duct.

■ KEY WORDS AND CONCEPTS

- Brush border
- Enterocytes
- Goblet cells
- Digestion
- Luminal or cavital digestion
- Contact or membrane digestion
- Unstirred layer of fluid
- Glycocalyx

- Passive diffusion
- Facilitated diffusion
- Active transport
- Starch
- Sucrose
- Lactose
- Maltose
- Amylopectin
- Lactase deficiency
- Endopeptidases
- Exopeptidases
- Trypsinogen
- Enterokinase
- Chymotrypsinogen
- Proelastase
- Procarboxypeptidases A and B
- Triglycerides
- Phospholipids
- Sterols
- Emulsification
- Carboxylic ester hydrolase
- Gastric lipase
- Pancreatic lipase
- Colipase
- Phospholipase A_2
- Cholesterol esterase
- Nonspecific esterase
- Micelles
- Critical micellar concentration
- Enterohepatic circulation
- Fatty acid–binding proteins
- Chylomicrons
- Apoprotein

■ BIBLIOGRAPHY

Ahnen DJ: Nutrient assimilation. In Kelly WN, editor: *Textbook of internal medicine,* Philadelphia, 1989, JB Lippincott.

Alpers DH: Digestion and absorption of carbohydrates and proteins. In Johnson LR, editor: *Physiology of the gastrointestinal tract,* ed 3, New York, 1994, Raven Press.

Ganapathy V, Brandsch M, Leibach FH: Intestinal transport of amino acids and peptides. In Johnson LR, editor: *Physiology of the gastrointestinal tract,* ed 3, New York, 1994, Raven Press.

Milne MD: Hereditary disorders of intestinal transport. In Smythe DH, editor: *Intestinal absorption,* New York, 1974, Plenum.

Rose RC: Intestinal absorption of water-soluble vitamins. In Johnson LR, editor: *Physiology of the gastrointestinal tract,* New York, 1987, Raven Press.

Solomon T: Pancreatic exocrine function. In Kelly WN, editor: *Textbook of internal medicine,* Philadelphia, 1989, JB Lippincott.

Tso P: Intestinal lipid absorption. In Johnson LR, editor: *Physiology of the gastrointestinal tract,* ed 3, New York, 1994, Raven Press.

Wellner D, Meister A: A survey of inborn errors of amino acid metabolism and transport in man, *Annu Rev Biochem* 50:911-968, 1980.

Wright EM, Hirayama BA, Loo DDF, Turk E, Hager K: Intestinal sugar transport. In Johnson LR, editor: *Physiology of the gastrointestinal tract,* ed 3, New York, 1994, Raven Press.

12

Fluid and Electrolyte Absorption

Leonard R. Johnson

Minerals and water enter the body through the intestine and provide the solutes and solvent water for body fluids. The electrolytes of primary importance include Na^+, K^+, HCO_3^-, Cl^-, Ca^{++}, and Fe^{++}. Each of these ions has one or more mechanisms by which it is transported across the intestinal epithelium. The purpose of this chapter is to consider these mechanisms and their relationship to water absorption and secretion.

■ BIDIRECTIONAL FLUID FLUX

During a 24-hour period 7 to 10 L of water enter the small intestine (Figure 12-1). Fluid derived from food and drink accounts for approximately 2 L. The other 7 L are derived from the secretions of the gastrointestinal (GI) tract: saliva, 1 L; gastric juice, 2 L; pancreatic juice, 2 L; bile, 1 L; and small intestinal secretions, 1 L. Of the amount entering, only about 600 ml/24-hour period reaches the colon, indicating that most water is absorbed in the small intestine. Because the average daily fecal weight is about 150 g, of which 100 g is water, 500 ml of fluid is absorbed daily from the colon. This volume represents 10% to 25% of the absorptive capacity of the colon, which is capable of absorbing about 4 to 6 L of fluid per day. Malabsorption of solutes and water

in the small intestine may result in enough fluid entering the colon to overwhelm its absorptive capacity and cause diarrhea. This, in turn, can precipitate severe electrolyte deficiencies. Although it is possible that ions and water may be added to the feces from colonic mucosa, the major source of water and electrolytes in a diarrheic stool is the small intestine (Figure 12-1).

It is evident from the foregoing account that several liters of fluid are secreted into the GI tract daily, and several liters are absorbed. The volume of fluid moving from blood to lumen (secretion) is less than that moving from the lumen to the blood (absorption), resulting in net absorption. Absorption generally results from the passive movement of water across the epithelial membrane in response to osmotic and hydrostatic pressures. Because of these so-called Starling forces, the consequent bulk flow of fluid is analogous to the flow of fluid across capillary walls. In the absence of food, ions are the most important contributors to osmotic pressure in the intestinal lumen. The ionic composition of the luminal contents may vary along the length of the intestine and is different from that in feces. However, luminal fluid generally remains isotonic with plasma because of the relative per-

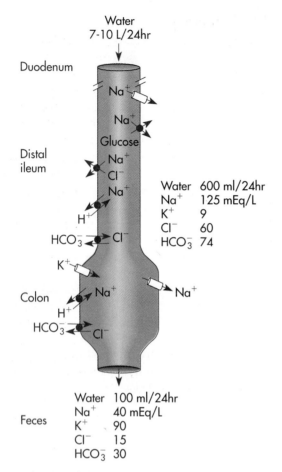

Figure 12-1 ■ Volume and composition of fluid in the small intestine and colon.

meability of the mucosal membrane. The continued production of solutes by colonic bacteria and the relative impermeability of the colonic membrane to water cause stool water to be usually hypertonic, 350 to 400 mOsm/L, to plasma.

■ IONIC CONTENT OF LUMINAL FLUID

Osmotic equilibrium with plasma of material entering the small bowel occurs rapidly in the duodenum. Water is absorbed from hypotonic solutions and enters hypertonic solutions. Na^+ and Cl^- also leave hypertonic solutions. Most of

this movement occurs through the relatively permeable junctions between the epithelial cells of the proximal small intestine.

Proceeding from the duodenum to the colon, the Na^+ and Cl^- concentrations in the lumen progressively become lower than the plasma concentrations. In the duodenum, Na^+ is approximately 140 mEq/L, equal to the serum concentration. The major anion is Cl^-. Sodium concentrations decrease in the jejunum and reach about 125 mEq/L in the ileum. The major anions in the ileum are Cl^- and HCO_3^-. Sodium decreases to 35 to 40 mEq/L in the colon, whereas the K^+ concentration increases to 90 mEq/L from 9 mEq/L in the ileum. The major anions in the colon are Cl^- and HCO_3^-.

These values indicate an effective absorption process for Na^+ that becomes increasingly efficient toward the distal portions of the gut. This is caused in part by a decrease in the permeability of the epithelium, preventing the back-diffusion of ions absorbed in the distal portions. Whereas the absorption of Na^+ in the distal gut is effective, the conservation of Cl^- is even more so. Chloride is exchanged for metabolically derived HCO_3^-.

Potassium is absorbed passively by the small intestine as the volume of intestinal contents decreases. The concentration of K^+ remains roughly equal to that in the serum (4 or 5 mEq/L). In the colon, net K^+ secretion occurs. Because of K^+ secretion and the exchange of Cl^- for HCO_3^- in the colon, prolonged diarrhea results in a hypokalemic metabolic acidosis.

■ TRANSPORT ROUTES AND PROCESSES

Ions move between the gut lumen and the blood by **transcellular** and **paracellular pathways** and by several processes. The passive movement of Na^+, both into and out of the lumen, is largely through the lateral spaces. This movement is regulated by the **tight junctions or zonnulae occludens**. The rate of this passive component is affected by electrochemical gradients and Starling forces. Normally these forces are small and account for only a small fraction of the net transport. They can, however, be altered under certain conditions, with marked effects.

The tight junction is about twice as permeable to Na^+ and K^+ as it is to Cl^-. Thus electrical potentials can arise across this structure. If, for example, NaCl is moving across the tight junction, the Cl^- will be retarded relative to the Na^+, and the surface toward which the movement is occurring will become positive relative to the other surface. Ions slightly larger than Na^+ and K^+ are much more restricted in their movement.

The pores through which transcellular diffusion takes place are probably larger (7 to 8 Å) in the proximal bowel than in the ileum (3 to 4 Å). This restricts the passive transport of solutes in distal gut and allows these solutes to exert a more effective osmotic pressure. In turn the reduced permeability makes carrier-mediated transport a more important contributor to net transport out of the lumen.

Na^+-Cl^- Transport

Physiologic models describing Na^+ and Cl^- absorption in the small intestine are shown in Figure 12-2. Sodium is absorbed from the lumen across the apical membrane of epithelial cells by four mechanisms. These include the movement of Na^+ by restricted diffusion through water-filled channels, the cotransport of Na^+ with organic solutes (e.g., glucose and amino acids), the cotransport of Na with Cl^-, and the countertransport of Na^+ in exchange for H^+. Because Na^+-Cl^- cotransport and Na^+-H^+ exchange are electrically neutral processes, the driving force for Na^+ to enter the cell is the Na^+ concentration difference between the luminal fluid and the cytoplasm. Sodium movement through pores and Na^+ cotransport with organic solutes are driven by the concentration difference and increase the negative electrical potential across the epithelial cell membrane. The contribution of restricted diffusion to overall Na^+ absorption is probably small, relative to other mechanisms.

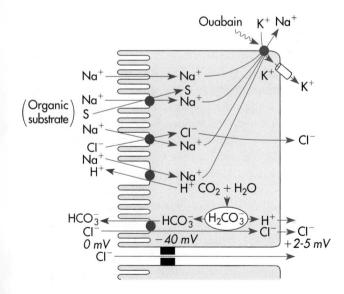

Figure 12-2 ■ Mechanism of NaCl absorption in the small intestine. Sodium enters passively, following the electrochemical gradient, by cotransport with nutrients such as glucose or amino acids, or by neutral cotransport with Cl^- or in exchange for protons via a countertransport process. Chloride is also absorbed by neutral exchange with HCO_3^-. Sodium exit from the cell is via the energy-dependent Na^+ pump, and Cl^- follows passively. The electrical potential difference across the apical membrane is −40 mV, and across the entire cell is + 3 to 5 mV with reference to the luminal side. Ouabain is an inhibitor of Na^+, K^+-ATPase.

The presence of these various mechanisms varies over the length of the small intestine. In the proximal bowel Na^+ is absorbed primarily coupled to H^+ countertransport and solute (amino acids and sugars) cotransport. In the ileum Na^+ is absorbed coupled to the absorption of Cl. Throughout the gut Cl^- is absorbed along the electrical gradient. In the ileum, coupled Na^+ transport is the major carrier-mediated pathway for Cl^- absorption. Exchange of Cl^- for HCO_3^- occurs in the distal ileum and increases dramatically in the colon and rectum. This mechanism accounts for the high HCO_3^- content and alkaline pH of stool water.

The Na^+-K^+ pump on the basolateral membranes of the absorbing epithelial cell maintains both the low intracellular Na^+ level and the negative membrane potential. Through this pump the Na^+ that enters by all four mechanisms described above is extruded into the intercellular spaces. The Na^+ pump is the well-known Na^+, K^+-activated adenosine triphosphatase (ATPase). This enzyme-carrier molecule is activated by intracellular Na^+ and extracellular K^+ to split adenosine triphosphate, releasing energy. In the process, three Na^+ ions are pumped out of the cell for every two K^+ ions pumped in. The pumping out of more Na^+ than K^+ entering creates a potential difference across the basolateral membrane, called an **electrogenic potential.** The pump is inhibited by cardiac glycosides (e.g., ouabain). Because Na^+ exit from the epithelial cell is coupled with K^+ entry, the intracellular K^+ concentration is much higher than the extracellular concentration. This causes the constant, downhill leakage of K^+ from the interior to exterior by K^+ channels on the basolateral membranes (i.e., the K^+ actively pumped into the cell returns to the exterior through passive leaks).

The epithelial absorption of Cl^- involves, in addition to cotransport with Na^+, countertransport with HCO_3^-. Production of HCO_3^- is by metabolic process taking place within the epithelial cells through the hydration of CO_2 by carbonic anhydrase. Both absorption mechanisms move Cl^- into the epithelial cell against an elctrochemical potential difference. The energy for the uphill movement of Cl^- is derived from the downhill movement of Na^+ into the cell or from the downhill movement of HCO_3^- out of the cell and into the lumen.

Because of the transcellular electrical potential difference—the serosal side is positive with reference to the lumen and with reference to the cell interior—Cl^- is driven passively from the cell and into the serosal fluid. Also, luminal Cl^- can move through the paracellular pathway into the serosal solution. The magnitude of this passive absorptive process is governed by the magnitude of the transmural potential difference (PD). That PD is developed through the action of the Na^+-K^+ pump and the absorption of Na^+ coupled to organic solutes. It is influenced by the resistance of the paracellular pathway to ion flow. In the small intestine the relatively leaky epithelium prevents the transmural PD from rising above 2 to 5 mV. In the colon, where the epithelium is less leaky, the PD is about 20 mV. Thus the driving force for Cl^- absorption is greater in the colon.

All regions of the colon absorb Na^+ and Cl^- (Figure 12-3). However, unlike the small intestine, the cotransport of Na^+ with organic solutes is lacking. Restricted diffusion is the primary mechanism for colonic Na^+ absorption. This electrogenic process, which increases in activity from oral to aboral regions, is dependent on channels that are under regulation by mineralocorticoids. For example, aldosterone increases the number of Na^+ channels and enhances Na^+ absorption. Sodium in the lumen of the colon also is absorbed through an electroneutral process that includes Cl^- cotransport. This probably involves Na^+-H^+ countertransport coupled with Cl^--HCO_3^- countertransport, as occurs in the small intestine.

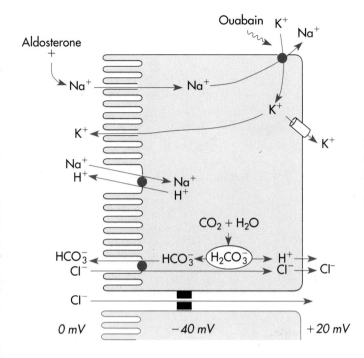

Figure 12-3 ■ Mechanism of ion absorption in the colon. Na^+ enters passively while Cl^- enters in neutral exchange with HCO_3^-. Net secretion of K^+ occurs.

A process of NaCl secretion exists in crypt cells of both the small intestine and colon (Figure 12-4). The mechanism involved is the neutral Na^+-Cl^- cotransport into the epithelial cells at the basolateral membranes. The energy required to drive Cl^- into the cell against an electrochemical potential is derived from the passive movement of Na^+ down its electrochemical gradient. The Na^+ that enters the cell is extruded by the sodium pump. Intracellular Cl^- attains high levels and diffuses across the apical membrane through selective Cl^- channels. These apical channels are relatively inactive under resting conditions but can be opened by an elevation in intracellular, cyclic adenosine monophosphate (cAMP) and/or Ca^{++}. These intracellular messengers can be elevated under physiologic conditions, as after a meal, by GI hormones (e.g., vasoactive intestinal peptide), neurotransmitters, and paracrine secretions such as prostaglandins. The intracellular messengers also may be ele-

vated to pathologic levels by exogenous agents such as bacterial enterotoxins (cholera toxin being the prototype).

The movement of Cl^- from the serosal to mucosal compartment polarizes the cell electrically, causing the lumen to become negative with reference to the serosa. This electrical potential difference causes Na^+ from the serosal fluid to enter the lumen via the paracellular pathway. Thus NaCl is secreted.

K^+ Transport

Diffusion through paracellular pathways in the small intestine is the primary mechanism by which K^+, derived from the diet or from secretions of the upper GI tract, undergoes net absorption. In the colon (but not in the small intestine) the apical and basolateral membranes are permeable to K^+. Thus, because of the high concentration of intracellular K^+ maintained by the Na^+-K^+ pump, some K^+ leaks passively across

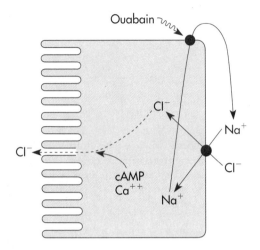

Figure 12-4 ■ Mechanism of NaCl secretion by the epithelium.

the apical membrane of epithelial cells. Factors that elevate intracellular K^+, such as aldosterone-stimulated Na^+ absorption, increase K^+ secretion.

■ MECHANISM FOR FLUID ABSORPTION AND SECRETION

Water absorption or secretion always occurs in response to osmotic forces produced by the transport of organic solutes or ions and can be explained in terms of a three-compartment model and local osmotic effects (Figure 12-5). In the absorbing intestine, solutes are moved from the lumen (first compartment) into and then out of the epithelial cell. This creates a local osmotic gradient, causing water to move from the gut lumen across the cell and into the intercellular space (second compartment). The entrance of water increases the hydrostatic pressure within this space, causing the bulk flow of water and solutes through the basement membrane into capillaries (third compartment). In the nonabsorbing intestine the imbalance of forces across the capillary wall leads to filtration of fluid into the interstitium. However, the capillary filtration rate is balanced by lymphatic drainage. In the secret-

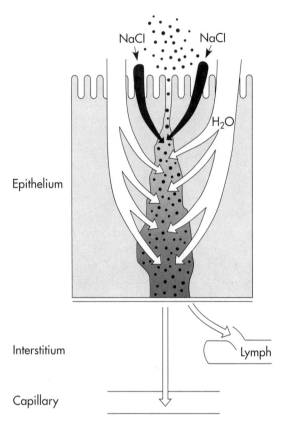

Figure 12-5 ■ Fluid absorption according to the standing osmotic gradient hypothesis. The sum of hydrostatic and osmotic pressures in the intraepithelial space, interstitium, and capillaries favors fluid absorption. In the nonabsorbing state, fluid filtering from the capillaries would be drained by the lymphatics. The attraction of fluid from the cytosol and interstitium because of high osmotic pressure in the lumen leads to secretion.

ing intestine, fluid in the interstitium is attracted osmotically into the lumen.

Osmotic equilibration, and therefore absorption, occur by different means in the duodenum and ileum. The duodenum functions to bring chyme into osmotic equilibrium with plasma. If a hypertonic solution is placed in the duodenum, isotonicity is reached by a rapid flow of water from blood to lumen, increasing the volume of the original solution. More distally, in the small intestine, absorption of solutes creates a gradient for water absorption. Thus the volume is decreased because of both solute and water uptake, and the isotonicity of the luminal solution is maintained during this process. In summary, the sequence of responses to hypertonic contents entering the intestinal lumen is, first, the dilution caused by osmotic attraction of water from the blood and then the movement of fluid from the lumen into the blood secondary to the transport of solutes.

If a hypotonic solution enters the intestine the flux of water from lumen to blood is greater than from blood to lumen, leading to net absorption of fluid. This in turn is followed by the isotonic uptake of fluid.

The gut normally absorbs all electrolytes and water presented to it and, unlike the kidney, does not appear subject to hour-by-hour homeostatic regulation. Nevertheless, some external regulation occurs. The autonomic nervous system has effects on NaCl transport. Adrenergic (α-receptor) or anticholinergic stimuli tend to increase absorption, but cholinergic or antiadrenergic stimuli tend to decrease absorption. Other agents (such as serotonin, dopamine, the endogenous opiates, enkephalins, and endorphins) alter gut transport, usually in the secretory direction. However, the opiates morphine and codeine increase gut absorption.

The ileum has relatively little ability to respond to Na$^+$ depletion and/or mineralocorticoids. By contrast the large intestine is sensitive to both these assaults that can increase Na$^+$ absorption and K$^+$ secretion. Mineralocorticoids can decrease the Na$^+$ concentration in fecal water from 30 to 2 mEq/L and increase K$^+$ concentration from 75 to 150 mEq/L. The influence of aldosterone on sodium transport is exerted at two points. There is an increase in Na$^+$ permeability of the brush border membrane caused by

the activation of new sodium channels. Also, aldosterone apparently increases the number of Na$^+$-pump molecules in the basolateral membrane.

Factors that cause the osmotic retention of water in the gut lumen or stimulate fluid secretion may lead to diarrhea. Saline laxatives such as epsom salts ($MgSO_4$) increase fecal water because of the slow and incomplete absorption of polyvalent ions. Disease states such as disaccharidase deficiency or monosaccharide malabsorption cause **osmotic diarrhea.** Cl$^-$ secretion that is stimulated by GI hormones and neurotransmitters following a meal is a physiologic aid to digestion. However, excessive Cl$^-$ secretion, with accompanying fluid secretion, may become pathologic in nature. Clinically the ability of the intestine to hypersecrete isotonic fluid is manifested in infections with bacteria such as *Vibrio cholerae* and *Escherichia coli.* The voluminous diarrhea is caused in part by failure of the absorptive mechanism, but largely is caused by the increased volume of secretion. Prostaglandins and VIP stimulate intestinal secretion in amounts comparable to those produced by bacterial enterotoxins. There is the additional suggestion that this secretory effect is mediated through cAMP because VIP, prostaglandin, and cholera toxin stimulate Cl$^-$ secretion in vitro, stimulate adenyl cyclase activity, and raise cAMP levels. The cAMP-stimulated Cl$^-$ secretory mechanism provides a focal point to pursue a physiologic explanation of **secretory diarrhea.**

■ Ca^{++} ABSORPTION

Absorption of Ca^{++} by the enterocytes is an important component in the regulation of whole body Ca^{++} (Figure 12-6). The transepithelial movement of the cation occurs against an electrochemical potential. The process, although not entirely known, is localized in the proximal small intestine. Calcium transport occurs in four major steps. First, Ca^{++} absorption involves entry at the

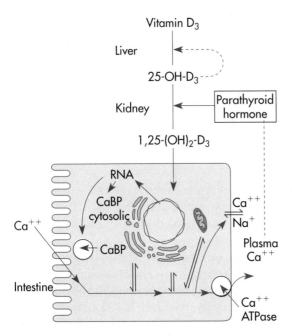

Figure 12-6 ■ **Calcium absorption by an entero-cyte within a larger scheme of Ca++ homeostasis. Vitamin D3, 1,25-(OH)2-D3, stimulates Ca++ transport by interacting with nuclear receptors to effect the synthesis of Ca++-binding proteins (CaBP). Ca++ enters the cell facilitated by brush border CaBP and exits via two mechanisms. It is speculated that CaBP in the cytosol stimulates Ca++-ATPase. Binding proteins in the Golgi, endoplasmic reticulum, and possibly mitochondria, prevent a rise in intracellular Ca++ during the absorptive process.**

erol) formed in the skin by the action of ultraviolet radiation on 7-dehydrocholesterol. Vitamin D_3 is transferred to the liver and converted to 25-OH-D_3. The kidney, through a step regulated by parathyroid hormone, converts 25-OH-D_3 to 1,25-(OH)$_2$-D_3. Enterocytes take up the 1,25-(OH)$_2$-D_3 where it reacts with a receptor molecule in either the nucleus or the cytosol (exact site unknown). The transcription of specific DNA and protein synthesis are mandatory steps in the action of 1,25-(OH)$_2$-D_3 on Ca++ transport. The Ca++ binding activity of the synthesized protein correlates with Ca++ transport. Presumably at least one Ca++-binding protein (CaBP) is inserted into the brush border and facilitates (gates) the entry of Ca++ down an electrochemical gradient.

Once inside the cell, CaBPs found in the Golgi apparatus and endoplasmic reticulum minimize the rise in intracellular free Ca++. It has been proposed, but not substantiated, that the mitochondria participate in this "buffering" action. This binding of Ca++ by the Golgi apparatus may possibly be a 1,25-(OH)$_2$-D_3-dependent process.

Exit of Ca++ at the basolateral membrane is against an electrochemical gradient and involves two mechanisms. The more important mechanism is the Ca++-ATPase, which may be 1,25-(OH)$_2$-D_3 dependent. The other is Na+-Ca++ exchanger, which functions when the Ca++-ATPase is saturated.

Calcium absorption is regulated over the long term by plasma Ca++ levels. As intestinal absorption of Ca++ rises, plasma Ca++ increases; this change inhibits the secretion of parathyroid hormone. In turn, formation of 1,25-(OH)$_2$-D_3 in the kidney is inhibited (Figure 12-6). A reduction in 1,25-(OH)$_2$-D_3 will eventually cause Ca++ absorption to wane, because the synthesis of new CaBP will cease. Although the mechanism of Ca++ absorption is not a closed issue, the model depicted in Figure 12-6 provides a currently popular working hypothesis.

brush border membrane. Second, a mechanism must be present to regulate intracellular Ca++ levels to prevent altered cell function. Third, **vitamin D** affects at least one of these steps. Fourth, Ca++ exit occurs at the basolateral membrane. In the remainder of this section a scheme compatible with these four points is presented.

Transport of Ca++ is initiated by 1,25-dihydroxyvitamin D_3 [1,25-(OH)$_2$-D_3]. This active product is derived from vitamin D_3 (cholecalcif-

■ IRON ABSORPTION

Absorption of iron is regulated by total body iron requirements and by the bioavailability of iron. Under physiologic conditions, dietary iron is acquired through transport processes in the proximal small intestine. Although the stomach, ileum, and colon have some capacity for iron absorption, this process is most prevalent in the duodenum and jejunum. Normally, because body iron is conserved, absorption of iron by the gut is low compared with the amount ingested.

Heme (derived from meat) is an important dietary source of iron. After it is absorbed intact by enterocytes it loses iron from its porphyrin ring. Heme is absorbed, probably by endocytosis, and digested by lysosomal enzymes to release free iron. In all other chemical forms, iron is absorbed only to the extent to which it can be released from food in ionizable form. The insoluble complexes of iron with food become more soluble at low pH. Gastric acid is important in solubilizing iron, and patients with deficient acid secretion absorb less iron. Organic acids such as ascorbic or citric reduce Fe^{+++} to Fe^{++}, which is absorbed more efficiently. Nonheme iron represents the largest fraction of dietary iron, and its absorption is dealt with in the ensuing discussion.

The cellular mechanism of iron transport has not been completely described. However, a working hypothesis can be synthesized from what is known about the influx of iron across the brush border, its intracellular processing, and its efflux across the basolateral membrane of enterocytes into the circulation (Figure 12-7).

The enterocytes of the proximal small bowel release an iron binding protein called transferrin, which binds two ions in the lumen. The transferrin-iron complex is recognized and bound by receptors on the brush border membranes of the duodenum and jejunum. The complex is absorbed, the receptor recycled, and the transferrin-

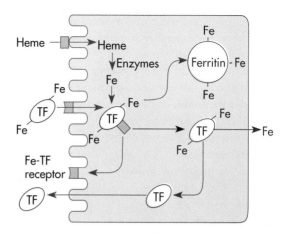

Figure 12-7 ■ **Iron absorption. Iron absorbed as heme is freed within the cell by an enzymatic process and bound to transferrin *(TF)*. Enterocytes secrete TF, which binds iron in the lumen. The complex is absorbed by a receptor-mediated process. Some iron is bound to ferritin and stored within the cell. Iron bound to TF enters the blood by an unknown process. The receptor is recycled and TF can be resecreted.**

iron complex is transported to the basolateral membrane. The iron appears in blood bound to plasma transferrin which is a β_1-globulin similar, but not identical, to intestinal transferrin. The movement of iron out of the enterocyte is poorly understood.

Some iron is transferred rapidly into the circulation while some is combined intracellularly with a specific protein, apoferritin, to form a complex called **ferritin.** A small amount of iron combined with ferritin can be taken up slowly by the body after conversion to free iron. However, most ferritin-bound iron is lost when the epithelium exfoliates. Iron transferred to the blood is transported through the cytosol to the basolateral membrane by a protein that conveys it to the intercellular space. The "transport protein" (intestinal transferrin) is similar to, but not identical with, transferrin. The latter is a β_1-globulin that binds to iron as it exits the enterocyte and transports it in plasma.

The body requirement for iron influences intestinal uptake. Absorption is thought to be regulated at a minimum of two sites. First, it depends on the binding of iron to brush border receptors, whose number is influenced by whole body iron requirements. Second, it is regulated by the ratio of intracellular transport protein to storage protein (ferritin). The formation of ferritin is greatest when the body iron levels are high. Thus iron transfer to the blood is low. The reverse holds during iron deficiency. For example, if iron depletion interferes with body functions such as hemoglobin synthesis, intestinal absorption of iron increases by the formation of more iron receptors on the brush border and by an increase in the intracellular iron transport protein relative to ferritin.

Systemic factors that control or regulate the rate of intestinal absorption of iron remain unknown. However, a feedback system has been proposed that entails both the transport and the storage of iron. Excess iron in the blood is carried to various body tissues, primarily the liver, where it is deposited as ferritin (storage iron), as in the intestinal mucosa. Ferritin-stored iron is in equilibrium with transferrin. During high storage conditions, transferrin in the plasma becomes saturated and can accept no more iron from parenchymal tissue stores or from mucosal cells. Thus iron absorption from the mucosa decreases. The existence of this feedback system and the factors that regulate the cellular mechanism of iron transport in the mucosa remain to be established.

■ SUMMARY

1. Approximately 9 L of water enters the GI tract per day. Of this amount 2 L are ingested and 7 L are secreted into the lumen. The small intestine absorbs about 8.5 L and the colon 0.4 L, leaving only 100 ml to be excreted in the stool.

2. The absorption of water occurs by diffusion down an osmotic gradient created by the absorption of Na^+, Cl^-, other electrolytes, and nutrients such as sugars and amino acids.

3. Four mechanisms account for the absorption of Na^+: passive diffusion, countertransport with H^+, cotransport with organic solutes (sugars and amino acids), and cotransport with Cl^-. The presence of these mechanisms varies along the length of the bowel.

4. Throughout the bowel, Cl^- is absorbed passively down its electrical gradient. In addition to being absorbed with Na^+, in the distal ileum and colon Cl^- is absorbed in exchange for HCO_3^-, which is secreted into the lumen and accounts for the alkalinity of stool water.

5. Crypt cells contain channels for Cl^- secretion in their apical membranes that respond to increases in cAMP. Various toxins, such as cholera toxin, and GI peptides, such as vasoactive intestinal peptide, trigger secretion via this mechanism, which depends on the Na^+, K^+-ATPase of the basolateral membrane.

6. The small intestine actively absorbs Ca^{++} by a process dependent on vitamin D, which stimulates the synthesis of a cytoplasmic Ca^{++} binding protein, and which in turn facilitates the entry of Ca^{++} across the brush border membrane.

7. Iron is absorbed as both heme and inorganic iron. A transferrin is secreted into the lumen by the intestinal cells. Transferrin forms a complex with two iron ions, which is absorbed by receptor-mediated endocytosis. Iron is released into the interstitial fluid and appears in the blood bound to a different transferrin.

■ KEY WORDS AND CONCEPTS

- Transcellular pathways
- Paracellular pathways

- Tight junctions or zonnulae occludens
- Electrogenic potential
- Osmotic diarrhea
- Secretory diarrhea
- Vitamin D
- Ferritin

■ BIBLIOGRAPHY

Binder HJ, Sandle GI: Electrolyte transport in the mammalian colon. In Johnson LR, editor: *Physiology of the gastrointestinal tract,* ed 3, New York, 1994, Raven Press.

Bronner F, Lipton J, Pansu D, Buckley M, Singh R, Miller A: Molecular and transport effects of 1,25-dehydroxyvitamin-D_3 in rat duodenum, *Fed Proc* 41:61-65, 1982.

Chang EB, Rao MC: Intestinal water and electrolyte transport: mechanisms of physiological and adaptive responses. In Johnson LR, editor: *Physiology of the gastrointestinal tract,* ed 3, New York, 1994, Raven Press.

Conrad ME: Iron absorption. In Johnson LR, editor: *Physiology of the gastrointestinal tract,* ed 2, New York, 1987, Raven Press.

Cooke HJ, Reddix RA: Neural regulation of intestinal electrolyte transport. In Johnson LR, editor: *Physiology of the gastrointestinal tract,* ed 3, New York, 1994, Raven Press.

Dharmsathaphorn K: Intestinal water and electrolyte transport. In Kelly WN, editor: *Textbook of internal medicine,* Philadelphia, 1989, JB Lippincott.

Powell DW: Intestinal water and electrolyte transport. In Johnson LR, editor: *Physiology of the gastrointestinal tract,* ed 2, New York, 1987, Raven Press.

Schultz SG: Cellular models of epithelial ion transport. In *Physiology of membrane disorders,* New York, 1986, Plenum Press.

Sellin JH and Desoigne R: Ion transport in human colon in vitro, *Gastroenterology* 93:441-448, 1987.

The Splanchnic Circulation

Eugene D. Jacobson

■ GENERAL CONSIDERATIONS

The splanchnic circulation delivers blood to and from the terminal esophagus, stomach, small bowel, colon, rectum, liver, gallbladder, pancreas, and spleen. The organs perfused by splanchnic blood vessels are intraabdominal structures, and all but the last mentioned have important digestive system functions. The splanchnic circulation contains several major vessels, including the celiac, hepatic, superior mesenteric, and inferior mesenteric arteries, and the portal and hepatic veins (Figure 13-1). The splanchnic circulation has three striking features, namely its **large blood flow, large reservoir function,** and the **diversity of organs** that it perfuses.

Blood Flow Values

The splanchnic circulation is the largest, systemic, regional circulation; that is, a greater fraction of the left ventricular outflow passes to the splanchnic viscera than to any other single region or organ of the body. Thus in an 80 kg adult male with a left ventricular output of about 7 L/min, blood flow to the splanchnic organs would approximate 2 L/min. The two largest branches of the entire aorta are the **celiac and superior mesenteric arteries,** each of which has a blood flow of about 800 ml/min. These two arteries provide 80% of the splanchnic inflow. The portal vein conveys about 1500 ml/min of blood flow from the stomach, small bowel, colon, pancreas, and spleen to the liver (Figure 13-1). Considered another way, in the resting adult human subject, the abdominal digestive organs comprise less than one tenth of whole body mass yet receive about 30% of the **cardiac output.** On a comparative basis, resting tissue perfusion values are about 0.1 ml/min per g tissue for the whole body and about 0.3 ml/min per g tissue for the splanchnic organs. Resting splanchnic perfusion values are augmented at mealtimes, especially in the mucosal lining of the hollow digestive organs and in the solid secretory organs (liver and pancreas).

The Reservoir Function

The reservoir function of the splanchnic circulation also exceeds that of any other region of the body. Thus the distribution of total blood volume in the resting person is such that the splanchnic organs contain one third of all the blood, with the remainder being located in all other body regions (Figure 13-2). However, when a person exercises, blood is squeezed out of peripheral sites and is directed into the heart and lungs. Of the

147

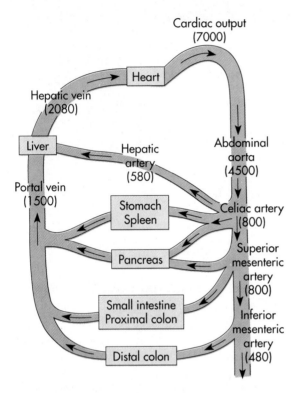

Figure 13-1 ■ The major blood vessels and the organs supplied with blood in the splanchnic circulation. Numbers in parentheses reflect approximate blood flow values for each major vessel in an 80-kg normal, resting, human adult subject. Arrows indicate the directions of blood flow.

blood volume that is so mobilized from all body regions, 70% comes from vascular reservoirs located in splanchnic organs.

The Diversity of Organs and Functions

The splanchnic organs exhibit a variety of functions including those that alter arterial inflow to the organs: increased gastrointestinal (GI) motility can enhance or reduce blood flow, increased secretion usually prompts an augmented blood flow, and an increased tissue metabolism is often associated with a rising blood flow. The celiac artery is a prime example of a splanchnic vessel

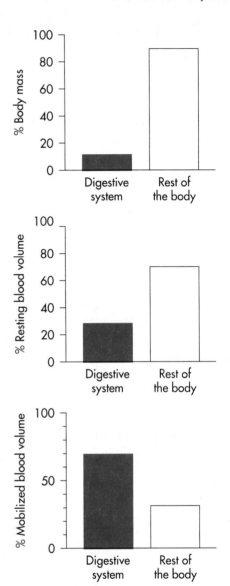

Figure 13-2 ■ Comparisons of the digestive system versus the rest of the body in terms of body mass, resting blood volume, and mobilized blood volume. The digestive system is the major reservoir of stored blood that has been mobilized to the heart in response to exercise and other stresses.

that serves various organs and tissues, namely the muscular walls of the stomach and duodenum, the glands of the gastric mucosa and pancreas, and metabolically active tissues in the exocrine pancreas, liver, and gastroduodenal mucosae. Response to a meal includes enhancement of all these organ functions, and the typical **circulatory response to eating** is an increase in both celiac artery and overall splanchnic blood flows.

■ HEMODYNAMIC CONSIDERATIONS

Three measurable parameters describe splanchnic hemodynamics and are related by the following equation (Figure 13-3):

$$\text{conductance} = \frac{\text{blood flow}}{\text{blood pressure gradient}}$$

Conductance is an estimate of the ease with which blood flows through the splanchnic circulation and is expressed in units of ml/min per mm Hg pressure. **Blood flow** is the volume of blood per unit time traversing the cross-sectional area in one plane of the splanchnic circulation and is expressed in ml/min. The **blood pressure gradient** is the difference between the mean systemic arterial pressure and the mean hepatic venous pressure expressed in mm Hg. For the splanchnic circulation, typical resting values would be as indicated by the following equation:

$$20 \text{ ml/min per mm Hg} = \frac{2100 \text{ ml/min}}{(110 - 5 \text{ mm Hg})}$$

The major vascular structures that regulate splanchnic conductance are the microscopic arteries and the arterioles, collectively known as the **resistance vessels** (Figure 13-4). The resistance vessels have diameters between 25 and 100 μm, and their walls are composed predominately of vascular smooth muscle (VSM). Because of their vast numbers, small changes in precapillary vessel wall tension are amplified rapidly into large changes in vascular **cross-sectional area,**

$$\text{Splanchnic conductance} = \frac{\text{Splanchnic blood flow}}{\text{Blood pressure gradient}}$$

$$\text{Normal flows:} \quad 20 \text{ ml/min per mm Hg} = \frac{2100 \text{ ml/min}}{(110-5) \text{ mm Hg}}$$

$$\text{Vasoconstriction:} \quad 10 \text{ ml/min per mm Hg} = \frac{1050 \text{ ml/min}}{105 \text{ mm Hg}}$$

$$\text{Vasodilation:} \quad 40 \text{ ml/min per mm Hg} = \frac{4200 \text{ ml/min}}{105 \text{ mm Hg}}$$

Figure 13-3 ■ The relationship between conductance, blood flow, and the blood pressure gradient across the splanchnic circulation. Conductance is the ratio of blood flow *(ml/min)* to the pressure gradient *(mm Hg)*, which would be approximately 20 ml/min per mm Hg in an 80-kg normal, resting adult subject. Assuming no changes in systemic arterial and hepatic venous pressures, splanchnic vasoconstriction would cause decreases in blood flow and conductance, whereas vasodilation would prompt increases in both parameters.

conductance, and blood flow. Thus when a chemical agonist (naturally occurring or a drug) binds to vascular muscle cell surface receptors to cause vessel wall contraction, there will be decreases in cross-sectional area, conductance, and blood flow through the vessels. This event might not prompt any rise in blood pressure and would be termed **vasoconstriction.** Some naturally occurring splanchnic **vasoconstrictor agonists** include angiotensin II, Ca^{++}, endothelins, norepinephrine, prostaglandin $F_2\alpha$, and vasopressin. Conversely, agents that elicit relaxation of splanchnic VSM cells prompt increases in cross-sectional area, conductance, and blood flow through the vessels without a change in blood

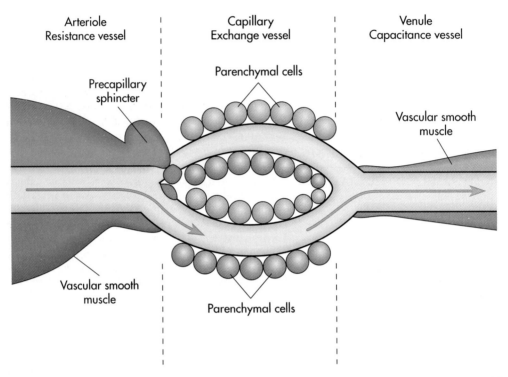

Figure 13-4 ■ Model of microcirculatory structures in the gut. The arteriole regulates most of the resistance to blood flow. The capillaries are the sites of chemical exchange between the blood and the parenchymal cells. The venule is the storage site for blood in the body.

pressure. These changes exemplify **vasodilation** and could be evoked by such naturally occurring **vasodilator agonists** as **acetylcholine** (ACh), adenosine, bradykinin, calcitonin gene-related peptide, histamine, nitric oxide, E- and I-type prostaglandins, substance P, and **vasoactive intestinal peptide** (VIP). The foregoing resting conductance equation can be used to describe a vasodilator or vasoconstrictor agent that makes a minute change in VSM tension leading to considerable changes in cross-sectional area, splanchnic conductance, and splanchnic blood flow (Figure 13-3).

■ **VASCULAR SMOOTH MUSCLE CELL TENSION**

When a VSM cell surface receptor binds an agonist (the first messenger) in the extracellular en-

vironment, cytosolic changes occur that lead to accumulation of intracellular **second messengers,** namely **cyclic adenosine monophosphate** (cAMP), Ca^{++}, or **cyclic guanosine monophosphate** (cGMP) (Figures 13-5 to 13-7). This form of signal transduction can proceed via three different intracellular cascades, each involving enzymatic activation that leads to increased concentrations of one of the VSM cytosolic second messengers. Multiple naturally occurring vasoconstrictor and vasodilator agonists have been cited above. Examples of second messenger generating enzymes include adenylyl cyclase, phospholipase C, and guanylyl cyclase. Adenylyl cyclase catalyzes cytosolic accumulation of cAMP (Figure 13-5). Phospholipase C hydrolyses membrane-bound phosphatidylinositol biphosphate into **inositol**

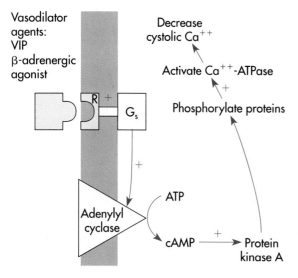

Figure 13-5 ■ Some vasodilator agents acting via VSM cell generation of cyclic adenosine-3′,5′-monophosphate *(cAMP)*. Binding of the vasodilator agent to its cell surface receptor *(R)* activates the stimulatory G protein *(G_s)* that turns on the catalytic subunit of adenylyl cyclase. This enzyme converts some adenosine triphosphate *(ATP)* into cAMP, which activates protein kinase A. The latter phosphorylating enzyme activates Ca^{++}-ATPase. Ca^{++}-ATPase extrudes Ca^{++} from the cytosol of the VSM cell into the extracellular space and the sarcoplasmic reticulum. Lowering the $[Ca^{++}]$ within the VSM cell causes vasodilation.

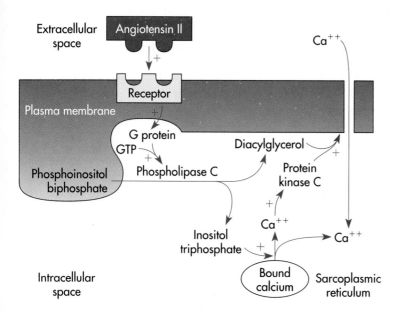

Figure 13-6 ■ Vasoconstrictor agents acting on VSM cells by increasing intracellular Ca^{++} concentrations. Receptor binding of a vasoconstrictor agent, such as angiotensin II, prompts receptor coupling to a G protein. The agonist–receptor–G protein assembly activates phospholipase C, which hydrolyzes phosphoinositol biphosphate in the cell membrane. Hydrolytic products (*inositol triphosphate* and *diacylglycerol*) are intracellular second messengers that act on different mechanisms to increase the intracellular $[Ca^{++}]$ and contract the VSM cell.

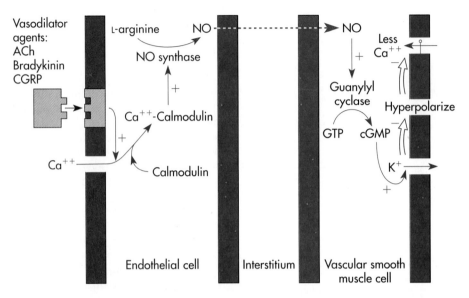

Figure 13-7 ■ **Another vasodilator cascade that involves nitric oxide *(NO)* and cyclic guanosine-3′,5′-monophosphate *(cGMP)*. Receptor binding of many vasodilator agents opens agonist gated Ca⁺⁺ channels in the endothelial cell. Ca⁺⁺ entering the endothelial cell binds to calmodulin, and this second messenger complex stimulates NO synthase conversion of L-arginine into NO. NO then diffuses from the endothelial cell into the VSM cell where NO stimulates guanylyl cyclase to metabolize some guanosine triphosphate *(GTP)* into cGMP. The cGMP increases the flux of K⁺ out of the cell through channels in the plasma membrane. The accelerated K⁺ loss hyperpolarizes the VSM cell plasma membrane *(inside negative)*, which closes the voltage gated Ca⁺⁺ channels, thereby decreasing the flux of Ca⁺⁺ from the extracellular compartment. The results are a decrease in the cytosolic [Ca⁺⁺] and vasodilation of the mesenteric resistance vessels.**

triphosphate and **diacylglycerol,** each of which elicits an increased VSM **cytosolic Ca⁺⁺** concentration (Figure 13-6). Guanylyl cyclase converts guanosine triphosphate into intracellular cGMP (Figure 13-7).

Ultimately the tension of VSM cells depends upon the cytosolic Ca⁺⁺ concentration, whose elevation starts the cascade of events underlying muscle contraction. The key chemical responses to an increased intracellular Ca⁺⁺ concentration involve activation of myosin kinase, adenosine triphosphate (ATP) hydrolysis with phosphotransfer to myosin, and the cyclic interaction of myosin and actin to contract VSM cells (Figure 13-8).

■ CONTROL OF SPLANCHNIC BLOOD FLOW

Multiple body systems are involved in the regulation of splanchnic blood flow, including the **cardiovascular, autonomic nervous, endocrine, paracrine and digestive systems** (Figure 13-9). Under normal operating conditions these different systems provide regulatory influences that are either additive and overlapping or opposing and counterbalanced. In some cases one regulator may be stimulated or inhibited by another in the manner of positive or negative feedback control. Examples of such regulatory mechanisms are discussed shortly.

When intracellular $[Ca^{++}]$ exceeds 10^{-6} M:

$$\begin{array}{c} Ca^{++} \\ + \\ Calmodulin \end{array} \longrightarrow Ca^{++}\text{-}Calmodulin \longrightarrow \begin{array}{c} \text{+ Inactive myosin kinase} \\ \\ \text{Active myosin kinase} \end{array}$$

$$Myosin + 2ATP \longrightarrow Myosin\text{\textasciitilde}(PO_4)_2$$
$$+$$
$$Actin$$
$$\downarrow$$
$$Muscle$$
$$contraction$$

Figure 13-8 ■ **Intracellular concentrations of Ca^{++} and VSM cell contraction and relaxation. When the cytosolic $[Ca^{++}]$ exceeds 10^{-6} M, Ca^{++}-calmodulin is formed, which activates myosin kinase, thereby leading to the phosphorylation of myosin and muscle contraction. When the cytosolic $[Ca^{++}]$ falls below 10^{-6} M, the foregoing steps are reversed and the VSM relaxes.**

When intracellular $[Ca^{++}]$ declines below 10^{-6} M:

$Ca^{++}\text{-}Calmodulin \longrightarrow Ca^{++} + Calmodulin$

$Active\ myosin\ kinase \longrightarrow Inactive\ myosin\ kinase$

$Myosin\text{\textasciitilde}(PO_4)_2 \xrightarrow{Phosphatase} Myosin$

Myosin and actin do not contract

} Muscle relaxation

Cardiovascular Control

General cardiovascular regulatory factors include those forces and their interrelationships that are designated as the cardiac output, the systemic arterial blood pressure, and the blood volume. Normal splanchnic blood flow depends upon a normally functioning cardiovascular system.

Dysfunction in the heart, great vessels, the peripheral microcirculation, or in the blood itself can cause a decreased splanchnic blood flow. Indeed, the splanchnic circulation is quite sensitive to a markedly diminished systemic arterial blood pressure or a decreased cardiac output, in part because survival of life in such situations requires maintenance of blood flow to the heart, brain, lungs, and kidneys at all costs. This dire need is met by splanchnic vasoconstriction and the redistribution of blood flow away from the digestive system.

An example of this type of cardiovascular dysfunction occurs during and following massive hemorrhage, say as a result of an automobile accident in which one victim suffers severance of a femoral artery with the loss of 2 L of blood. The results of such massive exsanguination include a cascade of circulatory events known as **oligemic shock** (Figure 13-10). The shrunken blood volume prompts a diminished venous return to the heart, which, by Starling's law, causes a decreased cardiac output and a drop in systemic arterial blood pressure. Arterial hypotension triggers pressoreceptor activation of the sympathetic nervous system. Sympathetic stimulation prompts release of catecholamines from vasomotor postganglionic fibers and from the adrenal medulla. The end result is diffuse vasoconstriction of the peripheral precapillary microvessels, especially those in the splanchnic circulation. The intensive splanchnic vasoconstriction, accompanied by the diminished arterial blood pressure and cardiac output, imposes an

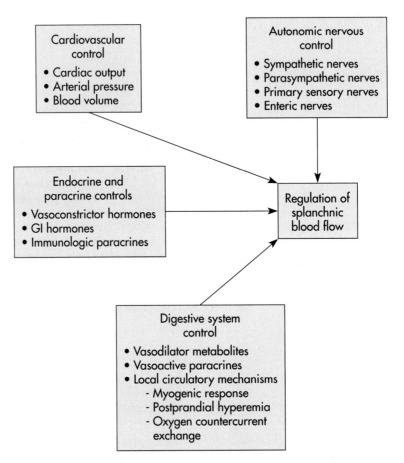

Figure 13-9 ■ **Major splanchnic blood flow regulators. Blood flow is controlled by cardiovascular, autonomic nervous, endocrine, paracrine, and digestive system factors.**

overwhelming **reduction in blood flow (ischemia)** and concomitant hypoxia on the digestive organs. If the **ischemic hypoxia** goes uncorrected for long, infarction of digestive organs occurs, usually in the small intestine, and will usually kill the patient.

Autonomic Nervous Control

There are four divisions of the autonomic nervous system (ANS) represented in the digestive organs, and their neurotransmitters are vasoactive substances (Table 13-1). The different divisions include the **sympathetic, parasympathetic, primary sensory, and enteric nerves.**

Sympathetic Nerves The adrenergic neurons include postganglionic efferent fibers that are projected mainly in perivascular neural sheaths surrounding visible arteries. These fibers terminate on the smooth muscle cells of precapillary resistance vessels (with diameters of 100 to 25 μm) where they release **norepinephrine** primarily. The catecholamine diffuses across the narrow synaptic cleft and binds to α_2-**adrenergic receptors** on the VSM surface. The binding

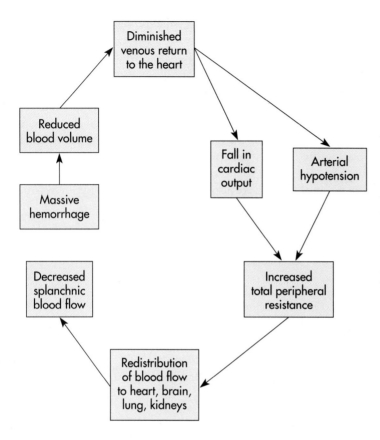

Figure 13-10 ■ The train of cardio-vascular system events leading from massive hemorrhage to diminished splanchnic blood flow. Oligemic shock due to blood loss causes successive dysfunctional changes, namely reduced venous return to the heart, decreased cardiac output and arterial blood pressure, increased total peripheral resistance, redistribution of blood flow away from the digestive system, and splanchnic ischemia.

T A B L E   1 3 - 1

Gastrointestinal vasoactive nerves and their neurotransmitters

	Neurotransmitter agents	
Autonomic nerve type	**Vasoconstrictors**	**Vasodilators**
Parasympathetic nerves		Acetylcholine
		VIP
Sympathetic nerves	Catecholamines stimulating	Catecholamines stimulating
	α_2-adrenergic receptors	β_2-adrenergic receptors
Primary sensory nerves		CGRP
		Substance P
		NO
Enteric nerves		Acetylcholine
		VIP

CGRP, calcitonin gene-related peptide; NO, nitric oxide.

step initiates the intracellular cascade that increases cytosolic Ca^{++} and constricts the resistance vessels of the splanchnic circulation (Figure 13-6).

Catecholamines also bind to **β_2-adrenergic receptors** on the smooth muscle surface, which initiates both the cAMP and the cGMP cascades (Figures 13-5 and 13-7). Increased intracellular concentrations of these two cyclic nucleotide second messengers cause vasodilation in splanchnic vessels. Therefore sympathetic neu-

rotransmitters evoke biphasic vasoactive responses, namely an abrupt, more striking decrease in blood flow followed by a more gradual restoration of blood flow, despite continued administration of norepinephrine (Figure 13-11). Other vasodilator agonists participate in the second phase of recovery from the decrease in blood flow, which has been termed **autoregulatory escape.**

Parasympathetic Nerves Cholinergic neurons are also extrinsic to the digestive organs, be-

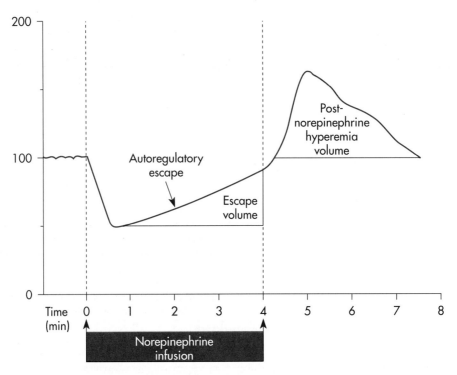

Figure 13-11 ■ The blood flow patterns during autoregulatory escape and postvasoconstrictor hyperemia. Although norepinephrine administration reduces intestinal blood flow initially, there is a gradual, partial recovery back toward the prenorepinephrine blood flow value, despite continued norepinephrine administration. One can measure the volume of blood flow occurring during escape from norepinephrine administration (the area under the blood flow curve labeled *escape volume*). The magnitude of escape in this example was about 80% of the blood flow before norepinephrine at the end of 4 minutes of norepinephrine infusion. Following cessation of norepinephrine administration there is a sizeable overshoot in blood flow. The magnitude of the hyperemia in this example is about 50% above the prenorepinephrine blood flow value.

ing mainly direct projections of vagal efferent branches and presacral parasympathetics. Some of these fibers synapse with sympathetic ganglion nerve cells, some with enteric cholinergic neurons in the myenteric and submucosal plexuses of the gut wall, and some with nonneural effectors such as visceral smooth muscle cells and blood vessel walls.

The primary parasympathetic neurotransmitters are ACh, VIP, and ATP. ACh binds to cholinergic receptors on the surface of endothelial cells. Receptor binding initiates the biosynthesis of **nitric oxide** and the cytosolic accumulation of cGMP in VSM cells (Figure 13-7). The end results are a reduction in the intracellular Ca^{++} concentration, a relaxation of the muscle, and vasodilation. VIP is also a vasodilator agent, but its intracellular effect involves mainly the buildup of

cytosolic cAMP. ATP is a mesenteric vasoconstrictor agonist probably because activation of contractile proteins for vasoconstriction is an ATP-dependent energetic process.

Primary Sensory Nerves These sensory neurons are small-diameter, afferent, C-fibers that also travel in the perivascular nerve sheaths, but in the opposite direction from sympathetic vasomotor fibers. Primary sensory nerves project from sensors in the mucosa or other gut wall layers and pass to dorsal root ganglia before entering the spinal cord. Primary sensory fibers also project from the gut wall directly to prevertebral sympathetic ganglia. Hence the C-fibers are able to inhibit the sympathetic impulse flow either at the spinal cord or sympathetic ganglion levels, thereby reducing vasoconstrictor input and increasing blood flow (Figure 13-12).

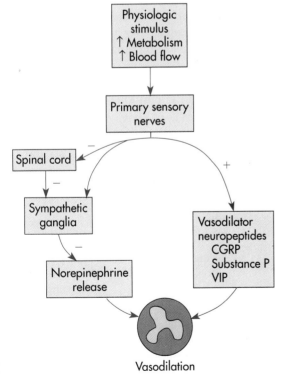

Vasodilation

Figure 13-12 ■ **Primary sensory nerve–induced vasodilation in the gut. Two mechanisms are involved in this vasodilation. Primary sensory nerve projections to the spinal cord and to the prevertebral sympathetic ganglion inhibit sympathetic vasomotor nerve release of norepinephrine. Primary sensory nerves also have efferent side branches that project to the intestinal resistance vessel. These fibers release vasodilator neurotransmitters such as calcitonin gene-related peptide (CGRP), substance P, and VIP. An arrow with a plus sign indicates a stimulatory effect, and an arrow with a minus sign indicates an inhibitory effect.**

In addition, some C-fibers pass directly from their mucosal sensors to gut wall blood vessels, where they release vasodilator neurotransmitters that increase blood flow. In this case an afferent nerve also has an efferent function; the phenomenon is termed **antidromic vasodilation** because the neural impulse flow to blood vessels is in the afferent direction (Figure 13-12).

The transmitters released by C-fibers are **neuropeptides,** the best known being **substance P, calcitonin gene-related peptide,** and VIP. Most of these neuropeptides are vasodilator substances that cause vascular muscle cell accumulation of cyclic nucleotides. Agents prompting release of these neuropeptides from C-fibers cause increased blood flow in the mucosal lining of digestive organs. Capsaicin, a chemical causing the pungent flavor of hot peppers and chilis, causes C-fiber release of neuropeptide transmitters, which evoke increased oral and gastric mucosal blood flow.

Enteric Nerves The enteric nervous system is comprised of dense neural networks located between the circular and the longitudinal muscle layers of the gut wall and between the submucosa and the muscularis propria. The nerve nets project fibers to glandular elements, visceral muscle cells, and blood vessels, as well as transmitting impulses via interneurons to portions of the network located at a distance further along the gut wall. The major neurotransmitter is ACh, although peptidergic and adrenergic transmitters are also released.

In summary, neural regulation of the GI circulation is complicated. There is an array of vasoactive neurotransmitters found in the four divisions of the ANS. However, the major first messenger governing vasoconstriction is norepinephrine released by sympathetic vasomotor fibers. Most of the remaining divisions and transmitters are vasodilator agents that operate to offset the initial effect of norepinephrine on blood flow.

Endocrine and Paracrine Controls

Endocrine messengers (hormones) are bloodborne substances that are released by source cells in one bodily location and then bind to receptors on the surface of target cells located elsewhere. Some hormones have direct vasoactive properties in the splanchnic region. Other endocrine substances alter blood flow to digestive organs by changing organ function and tissue metabolism.

Several hormones are vasoconstrictor agents in the splanchnic circulation (Table 13-2). These

T A B L E   1 3 - 2

Vasoactive hormones

Hormone	Source	Stimulus for release	Effect on GI circulation
Catecholamines	Adrenal medulla	Oligemic shock	Vasoconstriction
Angiotensin II	Renal JGA	Heart failure	Vasoconstriction
Vasopressin	Posterior pituitary	Oligemic shock	Vasoconstriction
Gastrin	GI mucosal G cells	Mealtimes	Vasodilation
CCK	Intestinal mucosal I cells	Mealtimes	Vasodilation
Secretin	Intestinal mucosal S cells	Mealtimes	Vasodilation

JGA, Juxtaglomerular apparatus; CCK, cholecystokinin.

include **catecholamines** released by the adrenal medulla, **angiotensin II** from the juxtaglomerular apparatus of the kidney, and **vasopressin** from the posterior pituitary gland. Normal blood concentrations of these agents are insufficient to alter blood flow to digestive organs; however, there are stresses and disease states in which their concentrations are elevated sufficiently to reduce GI blood flow. Examples of such conditions include the following: oligemic shock, heavy exercise, or a **pheochromocytoma,** which elevate circulating catecholamine concentrations; **congestive cardiac failure,** which is accompanied by increased blood levels of angiotensin II; and oligemic shock, which prompts rising plasma concentrations of vasopressin.

At mealtimes several peptide hormones are released into the circulation, such as **gastrin, cholecystokinin,** and **secretin.** These peptides stimulate a variety of digestive organ functions, namely gastric, pancreatic, and biliary exocrine secretion; propulsive contractions of the stomach and gut walls; active absorption of electrolytes, amino acids, and hexoses. These processes are energy dependent, and their stimulation elicits increased metabolism, which, in turn, increases splanchnic blood flow. The increased vascular perfusion makes available the substrates required for these enhanced digestive system functions, namely oxygen, hexoses, fatty acids, water, and selected electrolytes.

Cells of the immune system reside in close proximity to microcirculatory vessels of the digestive organs. **Mast cells** will cluster around the smooth muscle walls of resistance vessels in response to inflammatory stimuli and subsequently will degranulate, thereby releasing vasoactive paracrine substances such as **histamine** and **serotonin;** other immunologic cells release additional vasoactive mediators (e.g., cytokines, bradykinin, prostaglandins, and leukotrienes).

Digestive System Controls

The digestive organs influence their own blood flow. This form of vascular regulation involves metabolic, paracrine, and local circulatory mechanisms.

Vasodilator Metabolites As previously noted, mealtimes evoke increased digestive organ functions that enhance tissue metabolism and increase blood flow to support the augmented metabolic demand. When metabolic activity rises, there is increased local oxygen consumption and increased production of **vasodilator metabolites.** The decreased local tissue pO_2 and the increased concentrations of dilator amines, peptides, prostanoids, and adenosine relax the VSM walls of arterioles and precapillary sphincters. These microcirculatory hemodynamic events increase tissue blood flow and perfuse a higher proportion of capillaries. Since most diffusion of oxygen and nutrients from blood to tissue takes place across capillary walls, there is rapid replenishment of the substances required to maintain the elevated metabolic activity.

Vasoactive Paracrines Paracrine **substances** are produced and released by the cell of origin into the interstitial space. These agents then diffuse a short distance to reach receptors on the surface of nearby target cells, which react to the extracellular messenger. Some examples of vasoactive paracrine messengers have been identified previously as products of immunologic cells in the digestive organs.

Two other nonimmunologic, paracrine messengers that regulate blood flow to digestive organs are **adenosine** and **somatostatin.** The metabolic activity of any cell type involves the catabolism of ATP into lower energetic chemicals such as adenosine. Adenosine is a **vasodilator substance** in the splanchnic circulation. An example of physiologic vasodilation that is mediated by adenosine is the reciprocal increase in hepatic artery blood flow to the liver that occurs in response to a reduction in portal vein blood flow to the liver. This **hepatic arterial buffer response** maintains normal levels of liver blood flow when portal flow is jeopardized.

Somatostatin is a peptide that is produced by endocrine-like D cells of the GI mucosae. Somatostatin is released into the interstitium when gastric acid juice bathes the antral mucosal surface during mealtimes. Somatostatin inhibits nearby G cell production of gastrin and terminates the gastric phase of gastric acid secretion at mealtimes. Somatostatin also constricts gastric mucosal blood vessels and decreases local blood flow. The vasoconstrictive activity of somatostatin on digestive organ blood vessels has been exploited therapeutically to reduce splanchnic blood flow as part of the treatment of bleeding esophageal varices.

Local Circulatory Mechanisms Special vascular features of the splanchnic circulation constitute the third intrinsic digestive system regulator of blood flow. Two such mechanisms that have been described previously are autoregulatory escape (Figure 13-11) and hepatic arterial buffer response. Three additional local circulatory mechanisms are the myogenic response, postprandial hyperemia, and the oxygen countercurrent exchanger. These circulatory mechanisms occur mainly in the bowel.

The **myogenic response** of mesenteric arteriolar smooth muscle is independent of neuroendocrine influences. With this property of the resistance vessels, an increase in intravascular pressure stretches the muscular walls, which respond with an increase in tension. The result is that the augmented driving force of increased arterial blood pressure is offset by a decrease in cross-sectional area of the blood vessels. As the cross-sectional area is diminished, there is a decrease in vascular conductance. Since blood flow = blood pressure × conductance (Figure 13-3), the reciprocal changes in blood pressure and conductance maintain a steady blood flow. The myogenic response of resistance vessels also op-

erates to maintain a steady blood flow in the face of a decrease in blood pressure, in which case the muscular walls relax, thereby increasing cross-sectional area and conductance. Again there are reciprocal changes in blood pressure and conductance that serve to maintain a steady blood flow.

Postprandial hyperemia is the blood flow increase to a gut segment that occurs when a nutrient solution is instilled into the lumen of that segment. If isosmotic saline is instilled into the lumen, the increase in blood flow is minimal; if glucose is added to the saline solution, there is a larger hyperemia; and if an isosmotic saline solution containing micellar lipid (oleic acid + bile) is instilled, the increase in blood flow will be about 50% of the resting blood flow value (no instillation in the gut lumen). The mediator of postprandial hyperemia appears to be VIP released by the enteric nervous system.

The **oxygen countercurrent exchanger** is probably not important as a physiologic regulator of either normal tissue oxygenation or blood flow. However, in the pathophysiology of ischemia in the small intestine, this microcirculatory property aggravates the hypoxia and accelerates the necrosis of epithelial cells.

The villus is a finger-like projection of the small bowel mucosa that is about 1 mm long and 0.2 mm wide. In the core of each villus there is an inflowing arteriole that runs the length of the villus (Figure 13-13). At the villus tip the arteriole breaks up into a capillary network that lies deep to the superficial epithelial cells lining the villus. Oxygen crosses the capillary walls diffusing from red cell hemoglobin into the epithelial cells before the capillary blood flows into the villus venule. At the base of each villus, conditions are appropriate for another form of oxygen exchange. The arteriole and the venule are only 20 μm apart and their walls are permeable to lipid soluble substances like the oxygen gas, which is physically dissolved in the intravascular plasma.

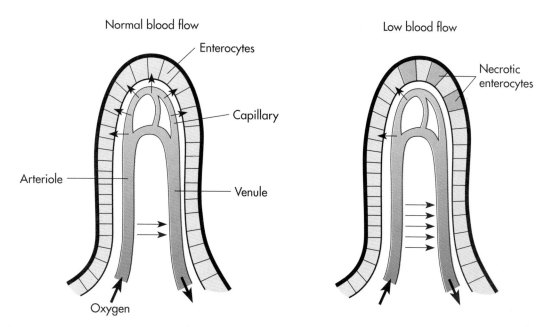

Figure 13-13 ■ **The oxygen countercurrent exchanger of the gut villus. When intestinal mucosal blood flow is normal, blood enters an arteriole in the villus core and passes to the villus tip. Here the arteriole breaks up into a capillary network. The capillaries convey blood beneath the epithelial cells that line the outside of the villus. The capillaries empty blood into the venule, which carries blood away from the villus to the body's general circulation. Oxygen is exchanged from red cells to epithelial cells only across the capillary walls. At the villus base the arteriole and venule are only 20 μm apart. Their blood flows are in opposite directions (countercurrent). This arrangement allows some lipid soluble oxygen that is physically dissolved in the plasma to shunt from arteriole to venule without reaching the capillaries. In intestinal low blood flow states (intestinal ischemia) this oxygen countercurrent exchange is exaggerated because of the slowed blood flow velocity. The shunting of oxygen away from the villus tip causes death of the epithelium at this site. Necrosis of villus tip enterocytes is an early pathologic finding in severe intestinal ischemia.**

Furthermore, the directions of blood flow are opposite in the arteriole and venule (**countercurrent flows**). Hence some oxygen diffuses from the arteriole, where the plasma oxygen concentration is higher, into the venule. Under normal conditions this shunting of arterial oxygen away from the capillaries is only a small fraction of the total oxygen that flows into the villus, and there is only a small oxygen gradient from the base to the tip of the villus (pO$_2$ of 15 versus 13 mm Hg, respectively).

The foregoing situation changes dramatically when the small bowel circulation is subjected to the insult of a **low flow state,** as in oligemic shock, nonocclusive intestinal ischemia, or with arterial occlusion due to a thrombus or embolus. In these ischemic conditions the oxygen countercurrent exchanger adversely affects oxygen availability to epithelial cells, especially those at the villus tips. Ischemia slows the velocity of blood flow through the villus, which permits a longer period for oxygen countercurrent exchange from the arteriole directly to the venule. This shunting of oxygen, which was innocuous under normal flow conditions, is imposed on a villus already suffering from severe ischemic hypoxia. The most adverse effect occurs at the villus tips, whose epithelial cells are metabolically the most active and, hence, most vulnerable to hypoxic insult. The **villus tip epithelial cells** are the first to perish and are sloughed into the gut lumen. Consequently, in severe ischemia of the small bowel, the initial evidence of mucosal necrosis on histopathologic examination consists of villi whose tips are denuded of epithelial cells.

■ PATHOPHYSIOLOGY OF THE SPLANCHNIC CIRCULATION

Blood flow to a splanchnic organ can be reduced abnormally or even brought to a halt by different pathophysiologic mechanisms occurring inside or outside the abdominal viscera. Some prominent disorders and events external to the digestive system that can cause ischemia of the bowel include recent cardiac surgery, septic or oligemic shock, acute respiratory distress syndrome, and subacute bacterial endocarditis (which showers emboli into the superior mesenteric artery). Disease processes intrinsic to the intestine that prompt severe mesenteric ischemia include thrombotic occlusion of a mesenteric artery, mesenteric venous occlusion, and **nonocclusive intestinal ischemia.**

About 25% of the cases of intestinal ischemia are classified as nonocclusive. This disorder tends to evolve more slowly than the gangrenous bowel resulting from an abrupt vascular occlusion taking place in thromboembolic diseases. In some ways this makes the pathophysiology easier to track and understand. Nonocclusive intestinal ischemia also bears a resemblance, in its pathogenesis and pathology, to other vasospastic, nonocclusive syndromes in the body that lead to life threatening infarction of the organ, such as coronary insufficiency and transient is-

chemic attacks of the cerebral circulation. In the case of nonocclusive intestinal ischemia the patient is usually elderly and suffering from coexisting serious cardiovascular disease such as **congestive cardiac failure** (Figure 13-14). The latter disorder is often treated with digitalis type of drugs. Heart failure causes a reduced cardiac output and an increased sympathetic nervous outflow. Digitalis enhances the vasoconstrictor action of norepinephrine on peripheral vasculatures such as the mesenteric circulation. Hence in these patients a low blood flow state already exists in the gut, and this state evolves into frank nonocclusive intestinal ischemia. Protracted ischemia causes **hypoxia of bowel tissue,** which is most marked in the metabolically more active mucosal epithelium and especially in the villus tips, where the countercurrent exchanger further robs oxygen from deficient cells (Figure 13-13). The severe injury and death of intestinal epithelium and the sloughing of cells exposes the mucosal parenchyma to the influx of luminal contents into the blood. Such materials are not normally absorbed and include many macromolecules, bacteria endotoxins and exotoxins, cellular debris, proteases and peroxidases, and electrolytes. Thus a **toxemia** is imposed on a dying patient with heart failure and bowel ischemia. Massive inflammation overwhelms the superficial mucosa as this area accumulates neutrophils and dying cells. Blood flow is further compromised by microvascular thrombi and vasoconstrictor paracrine substances such as endothelins, interleukins, leukotrienes, and platelet activating factor (PAF). The neutrophils turn their cytotoxic machinery loose upon the local parenchyma, and the mucosa fills with **necrotic cells.** Unless this situation is remedied with vasodilator drugs or surgical excision of the necrotic bowel, the hypoxic necrosis will extend through the gut wall and will cause peritonitis and death of the patient. Even with early diagnosis and aggressive treatment the mortality rate for

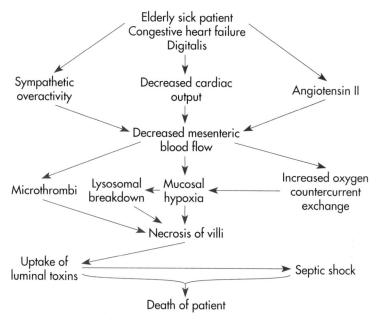

Figure 13-14 ■ **The pathophysiology of nonocclusive intestinal ischemia. The patient is usually elderly and has another serious cardiovascular disease, such as congestive cardiac failure being treated with digitalis. With this disorder and medication there is a reduced cardiac output and an increased resistance to intestinal blood flow prompted by sympathetic overactivity and release of angiotensin II. The decreased mesenteric blood flow evokes microthrombus formation and tissue hypoxia, the latter aggravated by the oxygen countercurrent exchanger. Intracellular lysosomes break down and release proteolytic enzymes. Mucosal necrosis ensues, most marked at the villus tips. With epithelial necrosis there is absorption of toxic substances from the gut lumen into the dying circulation. Septic shock follows with a usually fatal outcome for the patient.**

patients with nonocclusive intestinal ischemia exceeds 50%.

Finally, one has to inquire why protracted hypoxia is so poorly tolerated by cells. What pathophysiologic steps are involved in cell death during intestinal ischemia? The first step is conversion of the normal aerobic metabolism into an anaerobic state (Figure 13-15). The anaerobic conditions have two important consequences: (1) the intestinal mucosa contains ample amounts of the enzyme **xanthine dehydrogenase,** which is converted by hypoxia into xanthine oxidase, and (2) the normal aerobic cycle of ATP $\rightarrow$ adenosine $\rightarrow$ ATP is broken as adenosine accumulates and is further metabolized into inosine and then **hypoxanthine.** Ischemia is variable and occasionally there is reperfusion with more blood and oxygen. The oxygen plus hypoxanthine are converted into active oxidants by xanthine oxidase. Active oxidants include hydrogen peroxide, oxygen free radical, and hydroxyl radical; these compounds contain an additional electron in their outer ring and are highly reactive around cells. Active oxidants prompt lipolysis of cellular membranes, which causes increased permeability of the plasma membrane to Ca^{++}, K^+, and water. Active oxidants also cause circulating neutrophils to attach to the endothelium of blood vessels, especially in the venules. Neutrophils are capable of injecting

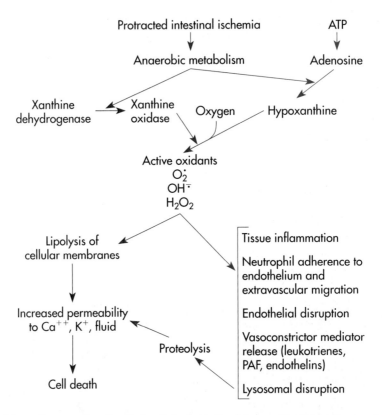

Figure 13-15 ■ **The pathogenesis of cell death in intestinal hypoxic states. Protracted gut ischemia imposes anaerobic metabolic conditions, which convert xanthine dehydrogenase to xanthine oxidase in the intestinal mucosa and which catabolize ATP to adenosine and then hypoxanthine. Xanthine oxidase metabolizes hypoxanthine and oxygen into active oxidants (oxygen free radical, hydroxyl radical, and hydrogen peroxide). These toxic oxidants provoke several adverse cellular responses leading to severe plasma membrane leakiness and cell death.**

toxic agents into endothelial cells (e.g., active oxidants, H^+, leukotrienes, and proteolytic agents). Then the neutrophils migrate between injured endothelial cells into the interstitium, where they injure parenchymal cells. The proteolytic enzymes released from lysosomes in injured cells also cause the plasma membrane to become leaky to ions and water. The influx of Ca^{++} and water and the efflux of K^+ are cytotoxic, and cells die.

■ **SUMMARY**

1. The three most striking features of the splanchnic circulation are the large blood flow, the large reservoir function, and the diversity of organs that it perfuses.

2. A greater fraction of left ventricular outflow passes to the splanchnic viscera than to any other single region in the body.

3. The splanchnic organs contain about one third of all the blood in the body.

4. The splanchnic circulation is important to digestive functions. The typical circulatory response to eating produces an increase in splanchnic blood flow.
5. Splanchnic blood flow is regulated by multiple body systems, including cardiovascular, autonomic nervous, endocrine, paracrine, and digestive systems.
6. At mealtimes, peptide hormones released into the circulation stimulate digestive organ functions, resulting in increased metabolism and increased splanchnic blood flow.
7. A variety of pathophysiologic mechanisms, including those related to and those external to the digestive system, can reduce or even halt splanchnic blood flow.

■ KEY WORDS AND CONCEPTS

- Large blood flow of the splanchnic circulation
- Large reservoir function of the splanchnic circulation
- Diversity of organs that the splanchnic circulation perfuses
- Celiac and superior mesenteric arteries
- Cardiac output
- Circulatory response to eating
- Conductance
- Blood flow
- Blood pressure gradient
- Resistance vessels
- Cross-sectional area
- Vasoconstriction
- Vasoconstrictor agonists
- Vasodilation
- Vasodilator agonists
- Acetylcholine
- Vasoactive intestinal peptide
- Second messengers
- Cyclic adenosine monophosphate
- Cyclic guanosine monophosphate
- Inositol triphosphate
- Diacylglycerol
- Cytosolic Ca^{++}
- Cardiovascular, autonomic nervous, endocrine, paracrine, and digestive systems
- Oligemic shock
- Reduction in blood flow (ischemia)
- Ischemic hypoxia
- Sympathetic, parasympathetic, primary sensory, and enteric nerves
- Norepinephrine
- α_2-adrenergic receptors
- β_2-adrenergic receptors
- Autoregulatory escape
- Nitric oxide
- Antidromic vasodilation
- Neuropeptides
- Substance P
- Calcitonin gene-related peptide
- Endocrine messengers (hormones)
- Catecholamines
- Angiotensin II
- Vasopressin
- Pheochromocytoma
- Congestive cardiac failure
- Gastrin
- Cholecystokinin
- Secretin
- Mast cells
- Histamine
- Serotonin
- Vasodilator metabolites
- Paracrine substances
- Adenosine
- Somatostatin
- Vasodilator substance
- Hepatic arterial buffer response
- Myogenic response
- Postprandial hyperemia
- Oxygen countercurrent exchanger
- Countercurrent flows
- Low flow state
- Villus tip epithelial cells

- Nonocclusive intestinal ischemia
- Congestive cardiac failure
- Hypoxia of bowel tissue
- Toxemia
- Necrotic cells
- Xanthine dehydrogenase
- Hypoxanthine

■ **BIBLIOGRAPHY**

Jacobson ED, Berguer R, Pawlik WW, Hottenstein OD: Mesenteric purinergic and peptidergic vasodilators. In Johnson LR, editor: *Physiology of the gastrointestinal tract,* ed 3, New York, 1994, Raven Press.

Granger DN, Grisham MB, Kvietys PR: Mechanisms of microvascular injury. In Johnson LR, editor: *Physiology of the gastrointestinal tract,* ed 3, New York, 1994, Raven Press.

Levine JS, Jacobson ED: Intestinal ischemic disorders, *Dig Dis* 13:3-24, 1995.

Review Examination

Select the Best Answer

1. If a peptide belonging to the gastrin/cholecystokinin (CCK) family and having a sulfated tyrosyl residue in the seventh position from the C-terminus is desulfated
   A. its pattern of activity will be identical to that of gastrin.
   B. no change in its pattern of activity will occur.
   C. its ability to stimulate gallbladder contraction will increase.
   D. its ability to stimulate gastric acid secretion will decrease.
   E. its pattern of activity will be identical to that of CCK.

2. Gastrointestinal (GI) hormones
   A. stimulate their target cells from the luminal side of the gut.
   B. are for the most part inactivated as they pass through the liver.
   C. are released from discrete glands within the mucosa of the GI tract.
   D. pass through the liver and heart before reaching their targets.
   E. are bound to plasma proteins in the blood.

3. CCK
   A. stimulates gastric emptying.
   B. is released by vagal stimulation.
   C. is released by protein and fat in the proximal small bowel.
   D. is released by distention when food enters the small bowel.
   E. is an important stimulator of gastric acid secretion.

4. Which of the following is *not* true about gastrinoma (Zollinger-Ellison syndrome)?
   A. Patients usually present with gastric ulcer.
   B. Patients develop diarrhea.
   C. Patients often have fat in their stools.
   D. The symptoms disappear following total gastrectomy.
   E. Following secretin injection the levels of gastrin in the serum increase.

5. Stimulation of an intrinsic nerve in the intestine causes contraction of an intestinal muscle cell through the release of which neurotransmitter?
   A. Acetylcholine (ACh)
   B. Nitric oxide
   C. Norepinephrine
   D. Somatostatin
   E. Vasoactive intestinal peptide (VIP)

6. A nerve ending that releases nitric oxide onto a smooth muscle cell of the jejunum is injected with a dye that spreads throughout the nerve. The nerve cell body labeled by the dye most likely will be located in the
   A. brain.
   B. celiac ganglion.
   C. myenteric plexus.
   D. sacral region of the spinal cord.
   E. thoracic region of the spinal cord.

7. A muscle cell that has no striations and has a ratio of thin to thick filaments of 15:1 most likely would be found in which region of the GI tract?
   A. External anal sphincter
   B. Lower esophageal sphincter (LES)
   C. Pharynx
   D. Tongue
   E. Upper esophageal sphincter (UES)

8. In the presence of drug X, application of ACh to a bundle of gastric muscle cells causes membrane action potentials, an increase followed by a decrease in intracellular free calcium, but no contractile response. Drug X most likely is inhibiting which step in the contraction-relaxation process?
   A. Activation of myosin light chain kinase
   B. Binding of ACh with membrane receptors
   C. Opening of membrane calcium channels
   D. Opening of sarcoplasmic reticulum calcium channels
   E. The spread of excitation among muscle cells

9. A lesion is made that results in loss of primary peristaltic contractions of the pharynx and esophagus; but secondary peristalsis of the lower esophagus occurs upon distention of the esophageal body. The lesion most likely is in the
   A. cortical region of the brain.
   B. cricopharyngeal muscle.
   C. enteric nerves.
   D. nucleus ambiguus of the vagus.
   E. pharyngeal muscle.

10. A segment of esophagus is removed and placed in a tissue bath. The circular muscle in the segment contracts tonically and relaxes upon stimulation of the nerves intrinsic to the segment. The segment is most likely from which region of the esophagus?
    A. Distal body of the esophagus
    B. LES
    C. Middle body of the esophagus
    D. Proximal body of the esophagus
    E. UES

11. A catheter that monitors pressure at its tip is inserted through the nose and passed an unknown distance. Between swallows it records a pressure that is subatmospheric and that fluctuates during the respiratory cycle, decreasing during inspiration and increasing during expiration. In which region is the catheter tip most likely located?
    A. Esophageal body above the diaphragm
    B. Esophageal body below the diaphragm
    C. LES
    D. Orad region of the stomach
    E. UES

12. A patient experiences gastric "fullness" after eating only a small quantity of food. Esophageal manometry reveals normal esophageal peristalsis but no receptive relaxation of the orad stomach. A lesion in which of the following is most likely responsible for the symptom and findings?
    A. The nucleus ambiguus
    B. The dorsal motor nucleus
    C. The vagus nerve trunk
    D. The enteric nerves
    E. The celiac ganglion

13. Contractions of the orad stomach, the proximal and distal antrum, the pylorus, and the proximal duodenum are monitored in a subject during the emptying of two meals that are identical except for their fat content. Compared with the low-fat meal, the meal high in fat would elicit

A. a decrease in force of pyloric contractions.

B. an increase in force of peristaltic antral contractions.

C. an increase in number of peristaltic antral contractions.

D. an increase in number of segmenting duodenal contractions.

E. an increase in number of tonic contractions of the orad stomach.

14. The electrical activities of smooth muscle cells of the orad stomach, the proximal and distal antrum, and the proximal duodenum are monitored in a fasted subject. Compared with the period of minimal contractions, the period of intense contractions of the migrating motor complex is characterized by

A. a decrease in apparent propagation velocity of antral slow waves.

B. a decrease in frequency of duodenal slow waves.

C. an increase in amplitude of antral slow waves.

D. an increase in frequency of antral slow waves.

E. the occurrence of slow waves in the orad stomach.

15. Compared with the gastric motility response to a meal in an individual with intact vagus nerves, the response in an individual whose vagus nerves have been cut at a level just above the diaphragm would be characterized by

A. decreased emptying rate of liquids.

B. decreased emptying rate of solids.

C. increased accommodation of the meal.

D. increased mechanical reduction of food particle size.

E. increased mixing of contents.

16. Which of the following procedures would decrease the rate of gastric emptying of a mixed meal of solid foods and liquids?

A. Application of a local anesthetic to the duodenal mucosa

B. Application of a local anesthetic to the gastric mucosa

C. Infusion of an isotonic solution of sodium bicarbonate into the duodenum

D. Infusion of an isotonic solution of sodium chloride into the stomach

E. Infusion of an isotonic solution of sodium oleate into the duodenum

17. A patient experiences a rapid rate of transit of contents from the duodenum to the cecum. What characteristic would contractions recorded at various loci of the small intestine exhibit during this time?

A. A frequency greater than that of the slow wave

B. Low in force

C. Mostly peristaltic

D. Mostly segmenting

E. Mostly tonic

18. Intravenous injection of a hormone initiates a phase of intense sequential contractions of the proximal duodenum that appears to migrate slowly toward the cecum. Which hormone was most likely injected?

A. CCK

B. Gastrin

C. Motilin

D. Secretin

E. VIP

19. A region of the intestine contracts weakly upon stimulation of its extrinsic nerves. Distention of the region elicits a peristaltic reflex, but with weak contractions. Slow wave activity is absent. Taken together, these findings suggest a disorder of the

A. enteric nerves.

B. parasympathetic nerves.

C. release of motilin.

D. smooth muscle cells.

E. sympathetic nerves.

20. The electrical activity of the musculature is monitored at two loci, A and B, of the small intestine. Over a period of one minute, 12 slow waves occur at locus A and eight slow waves occur at locus B. Spike potentials are superimposed on four of the slow waves at locus A and on six of the slow waves at locus B. Analysis of these data suggest that
    A. locus B is orad to locus A.
    B. segmenting contractions were occurring at locus A while peristaltic contractions were occurring at locus B during that 1 minute.
    C. the duration of each contraction at locus A was longer than the duration of each contraction at locus B during that 1 minute.
    D. the force of each contraction at locus A was greater than the force of each contraction at locus B during that 1 minute.
    E. the number of contractions at locus B was greater than the number of contractions at locus A during that 1 minute.

21. Intraluminal pressure is monitored from a region of colon that exhibits a relatively constant resting pressure of about 20 mm Hg. When an adjacent region of colon is distended, resting pressure falls to near 0 and then increases slowly back toward 20 mm Hg even though the distention persists. The region being monitored is most likely the
    A. ascending colon.
    B. external anal sphincter.
    C. ileocecal sphincter.
    D. internal anal sphincter.
    E. transverse colon.

22. Characteristics of segmental contractions include
    A. increased frequency of occurrence in response to increased circulating levels of epinephrine.
    B. occurrence at a frequency higher than that for peristaltic contractions.
    C. occurrence at a frequency that is higher in the sigmoid colon than in the rectum.
    D. occurrence at a frequency that is higher than that for slow waves in the same region.
    E. the loss of haustral markings when segmental contractions are occurring.

23. Intraluminal pressure is monitored from a region of colon that exhibits a stable resting pressure of about 20 mm Hg. When the hormone gastrin is injected, resting pressure falls toward 0 for several seconds before increasing slowly back toward 20 mm Hg. The region being monitored is most likely the
    A. ascending colon.
    B. external anal sphincter.
    C. ileocecal sphincter.
    D. internal anal sphincter.
    E. transverse colon.

24. In a patient in whom resting tone of the internal anal sphincter is normal, distention of the rectum induces normal relaxation of the internal anal sphincter, no change in tone of the external anal sphincter, and no sensation of the urge to defecate. These findings are consistent with the finding of damage to the
    A. enteric nerves.
    B. internal anal sphincter.
    C. pudendal nerves.
    D. spinal cord.
    E. transverse colon.

25. The digestive action of saliva on starch is due to
    A. lactoferrin.
    B. lingual lipase.
    C. ptyalin.
    D. kallikrein.
    E. bradykinin.
26. At high rates of secretion, compared with low rates, saliva would have a lower concentration of
    A. Na^+.
    B. water.
    C. Cl^-.
    D. HCO_3^-.
27. All of the following are characteristic of saliva *except that*
    A. it has a high K^+ concentration.
    B. there is a large volume of secretion relative to the weight of the glands.
    C. both parasympathetic and sympathetic stimulation increase its flow.
    D. it is hypotonic.
    E. it is primarily regulated by hormones.
28. Salivary secretion is inhibited by
    A. smell.
    B. taste.
    C. nausea.
    D. pressure of food in mouth.
    E. sleep.
29. Which of the following substances or combinations will produce the highest rate of acid secretion?
    Each compound is given at its half maximal dose.
    A. Histamine
    B. Gastrin
    C. Gastrin plus secretin
    D. ACh
    E. Histamine plus gastrin

30. Acid secretion during the cephalic response to a meal
    A. fails to occur when the antrum is acidified.
    B. is triggered by the entrance of food into the stomach.
    C. is prevented by vagotomy.
    D. is inhibited by insulin injection.
    E. is stimulated only by ACh acting on the parietal cells.
31. Following the administration of histamine to a fasting individual, all of the following will occur within the parietal cells *except*
    A. a decreased amount of tubulovesicles.
    B. increased carbonic anhydrase activity.
    C. increased H^+, K^+-ATPase activity.
    D. an increased number of mitochondria.
    E. an increased area devoted to the intracellular canaliculus.
32. According to the two-component hypothesis for gastric acid secretion, the H^+ concentration in gastric secretion increases with the rate of secretion because
    A. the volume of the oxyntic component increases.
    B. the concentration of H^+ being secreted by the parietal cells increases.
    C. the volume of the nonoxyntic component decreases.
    D. the secretion of Na^+ is inhibited.
    E. the secretion becomes hypertonic.
33. Antral gastrin release is stimulated by all of the following *except*
    A. bombesin gastrin-releasing peptide.
    B. ACh.
    C. fat in the stomach.
    D. protein digestion products in the stomach.
    E. distention of the antrum.

34. The presence of acid (pH <3) in the duodenum
    A. inhibits gastrin release via somatostatin.
    B. increases pancreatic bicarbonate secre-
    tion.
    C. decreases bile production.
    D. increases gastric acid secretion.
    E. inhibits pancreatic enzyme secretion.
35. In someone with a total absence of gastric
parietal cells, one would expect to find each
of the following *except*
    A. decreased digestion of dietary protein.
    B. decreased absorption of vitamin B_{12}.
    C. little or no pepsin activity.
    D. increased growth of gut bacteria.
    E. lower than normal pancreatic bicarbon-
    ate secretion.
36. Administration of a drug that blocks the H^+,
K^+-ATPase of the parietal cells of a secreting
stomach
    A. will have no effect on the volume of se-
    cretion.
    B. will increase the concentration of H^+ in
    the secretion.
    C. will decrease the concentration of Na^+ in
    the secretion.
    D. will decrease the pH of the gastric venous
    blood.
    E. will decrease the potential difference
    across the stomach.
37. The interruption of vagal afferent fibers from
the stomach would
    A. decrease the acid secretory response to
    sham-feeding.
    B. decrease the release of gastrin by digested
    protein.
    C. decrease acid secretion in response to dis-
    tention.
    D. decrease the release of somatostatin.
    E. increase acid secretion in response to his-
    tamine.

38. Between meals when the stomach is empty
of food
    A. it contains a large volume of juice with
    pH approximately equal to 5.
    B. gastrin release is inhibited by a strongly
    acidic solution.
    C. it contains a small volume of gastric juice
    with a pH near neutrality.
    D. bombesin acts on the parietal cells to in-
    hibit secretion.
    E. it secretes large volumes of weakly acidic
    juice.
39. During the cephalic phase
    A. secretin stimulates pepsin secretion.
    B. CCK stimulates pancreatic enzyme secre-
    tion.
    C. ACh stimulates the G-cell to release gas-
    trin.
    D. bombesin stimulates parietal cell secre-
    tion.
    E. ACh stimulates pancreatic enzyme secre-
    tion.
40. In humans maximal rates of pancreatic bicarbonate secretion in response to a meal
are due to
    A. the effects of small amounts of secretin
    being potentiated by ACh and CCK.
    B. large amounts of secretin released from
    the duodenal mucosa.
    C. VIP acting on the ductule cells.
    D. potentiation between CCK and ACh re-
    leased from vagovagal reflexes.
    E. potentiation between small amounts of
    secretin and gastrin.
41. Vagal stimulation
    A. potentiates the effect of CCK on pancre-
    atic acinar cells.
    B. directly stimulates pancreatic enzyme se-
    cretion.
    C. releases CCK from the duodenal mucosa.
    D. inhibits the effect of secretin on pancre-
    atic ductule cells.
    E. releases secretin from duodenal mucosa.

42. Pancreatic enzyme secretion
    A. contains enzymes for the digestion of fat and protein but not carbohydrate.
    B. is primarily stimulated by secretin.
    C. is stimulated by pancreatic polypeptide.
    D. originates from the ductule cells.
    E. occurs primarily during the intestinal phase of the secretory response.

43. Pancreatic bicarbonate
    A. is secreted primarily from acinar cells.
    B. is secreted in quantities approximately equal to those of gastric acid.
    C. is stimulated primarily during the gastric phase of digestion.
    D. secretion causes an increase in the pH of pancreatic venous blood.
    E. ion concentrations in pancreatic juice decrease with increasing rates of volume secretion.

44. Pancreatic enzymes
    A. are synthesized in response to a secretory stimulus.
    B. are stored in Golgi vesicles.
    C. are secreted in response to carbohydrate in the duodenum.
    D. are secreted in response to sham-feeding.
    E. are involved in the breakdown of disaccharides.

45. A sample of bile taken from the gallbladder is compared with a sample of bile collected as it is being secreted from the liver. Compared with hepatic bile, the gallbladder bile will differ in that its
    A. bile salt concentration will be less.
    B. cholesterol/bile salt ratio will be greater.
    C. osmolality will be greater.
    D. phospholipid concentration will be less.
    E. sodium concentration will be greater.

46. Bile acid A has a greater solubility in intestinal fluid than does bile acid B. Compared with bile acid B, bile acid A is more likely to be
    A. a secondary bile acid.
    B. a trihydroxy rather than a dihydroxy bile acid.
    C. absorbed passively in the jejunum.
    D. unconjugated.
    E. undissociated.

47. When the distal ileum is removed, there will be an increase in bile acid
    A. levels in hepatic venous blood.
    B. levels in portal venous blood.
    C. secretion by hepatocytes.
    D. storage in the gallbladder.
    E. synthesis by hepatocytes.

48. As the bile that is secreted by the hepatocytes flows through the hepatic ducts on the way to the gallbladder, there is an increase in bile
    A. bicarbonate concentration.
    B. bilirubin content.
    C. chloride concentration.
    D. hydrogen ion concentration.
    E. osmolality.

49. The rate of absorption of free galactose in the small intestine, initially occurring at a submaximal rate, would be
    A. increased by adding an equal amount of glucose to the lumen.
    B. decreased by adding amino acids to the lumen.
    C. decreased by adding fructose to the lumen.
    D. increased by the addition of trehalose to the lumen.
    E. decreased by hypoxia in the enterocytes.

50. Which of the following enzymes is located in the brush border and plays a role in protein digestion?
    A. α-dextrinase
    B. Carboxypeptidase A
    C. Pepsin
    D. Enterokinase
    E. Lactase

51. Colipase facilitates fat assimilation by
    A. digesting triglycerides.
    B. transporting fatty acids across cell membranes.
    C. preventing the inactivation of lipase by bile salts.
    D. converting prolipase to lipase.
    E. binding fatty acids and monoglycerides after they have been absorbed by the enterocytes.

52. Most medium-chain fatty acids do not appear in chylomicrons because
    A. they are not absorbed by enterocytes.
    B. they are not transported by fatty acid–binding proteins.
    C. they do not bind to apoproteins.
    D. triglycerides containing them are not digested by pancreatic lipase.
    E. they are absorbed directly into the blood.

53. In the absence of enterokinase one would also expect a decrease in the activity of
    A. pepsin.
    B. lipase.
    C. chymotrypsin.
    D. amylase.
    E. sucrase.

54. Amino acids
    A. are primarily absorbed in the distal gut.
    B. are, for the most part, absorbed by passive mechanisms.
    C. compete with glucose for Na^+ during their absorption.
    D. appear in the blood more rapidly when presented to the gut as small peptides rather than as free amino acids.
    E. are produced in the lumen primarily by the action of endopeptidases.

55. Each of the following acts as a good emulsifying agent *except*
    A. cholesterol.
    B. bile salts.
    C. fatty acids.
    D. lecithin.
    E. dietary protein.

56. Colipase
    A. digests the ester link in 2-monoglycerides.
    B. is a brush border enzyme.
    C. has no enzymatic activity.
    D. lowers the pH optimum of pancreatic lipase to match that of duodenal contents.
    E. displaces pancreatic lipase from the surface of emulsion droplets.

57. The fact that patients with a congenital absence of one of the amino acid carriers do not become deficient in that amino acid is due to the fact that
    A. the amino acid is absorbed by passive diffusion.
    B. the amino acid can make use of other carriers.
    C. the amino acid is absorbed by facilitated diffusion.
    D. peptides containing the amino acid are absorbed by different carriers.
    E. the amino acid is an essential amino acid.

58. Within the enterocytes
    A. triglycerides are resynthesized in the smooth endoplasmic reticulum.
    B. chylomicrons are synthesized in the smooth endoplasmic reticulum.
    C. fatty acid–binding protein transports long-chain fatty acids to the Golgi apparatus.
    D. triglycerides are synthesized from medium- and short-chain fatty acids.
    E. the major triglyceride resynthesis pathway makes use of dietary glycerol.

59. Of the 8 to 10 L of H_2O entering the digestive tract per day
    A. only 100 to 200 ml are excreted in the stool.
    B. most comes from the diet (includes liquids).
    C. most is absorbed in the large intestine.
    D. gastric secretions contribute twice the volume of those from the pancreas.
    E. most is absorbed against its own concentration gradient.

60. In the small intestine Na^+ is absorbed by each of the following processes *except*
    A. diffusion.
    B. coupled to amino acid absorption.
    C. coupled to galactose absorption.
    D. coupled to the transport of H^+ in the opposite direction.
    E. coupled to the absorption of HCO_3^-.

61. In the distal portion of the ileum
    A. most fatty acids are absorbed.
    B. Cl^- is absorbed in exchange for HCO_3^-.
    C. Na^+ absorption occurs primarily coupled to glucose and amino acids.
    D. intrinsic factor is secreted.
    E. K^+ is absorbed in exchange for Na^+.

62. In the small intestine each of the following is true regarding Cl^- absorption *except that*
    A. it occurs down its electrical gradient.
    B. it occurs in exchange for Na^+.
    C. it occurs in exchange for HCO_3^-.
    D. it will result in the absorption of water.
    E. it occurs along the entire length of small bowel.

63. Osmotic diarrhea may be the result of each of the following *except*
    A. cholera.
    B. lactase deficiency.
    C. inactivation of pancreatic lipase.
    D. Zollinger-Ellison syndrome (gastrinoma).
    E. loss of mucosal surface area in the small intestine.

64. Secretion of Cl^- by the small intestine
    A. occurs in exchange for HCO_3^-.
    B. takes place primarily in the villous cells.
    C. is inhibited by ouabain.
    D. produces an osmotic diarrhea.
    E. depends on an adenosine triphosphatase in the brush border membrane.

65. In the splanchnic circulation
    A. portal vein blood flow exceeds hepatic vein blood flow by about 50%.
    B. portal vein blood flow exceeds hepatic artery blood flow by about 50%.
    C. celiac artery blood flow exceeds hepatic vein blood flow by about 50%.
    D. celiac artery blood flow exceeds hepatic artery blood flow by about 50%.
    E. hepatic vein blood flow exceeds hepatic artery blood flow by about 50%.

66. The digestive system
    A. weighs more than the rest of the body.
    B. weighs half as much as the rest of the body.
    C. stores more blood that can be mobilized during exercise than any other part of the body.
    D. stores less blood that can be mobilized during exercise than do the voluntary muscles.
    E. contains half of the resting blood volume in the entire body.

67. Splanchnic conductance
    A. equals the blood pressure gradient ÷ splanchnic blood flow.
    B. increases during vasodilation.
    C. decreases during vasodilation.
    D. increases during vasoconstriction.
    E. decreases when splanchnic blood flow increases and the pressure gradient remains unchanged.

68. The major function of
    A. arterioles is to permit oxygen exchange from blood to parenchymal cells.
    B. arterioles is to permit glucose exchange from blood to parenchymal cells.
    C. venules is to provide resistance to the flow of blood.
    D. venules is to store blood that can be mobilized during exercise and other stresses.
    E. capillaries is to offer resistance to blood flow.

69. Vasodilator agents that bind to vascular smooth muscle surface receptors
    A. decrease the cytosolic calcium concentration.
    B. decrease the cytosolic cyclic adenosine monophosphate concentration.
    C. decrease the cytosolic cyclic guanosine monophosphate concentration.
    D. increase calcium flux into the cytosol from the extracellular space.
    E. increase calcium release from the sarcoplasmic reticulum.

70. A vasoconstrictor agent such as angiotensin II
    A. activates phospholipase C hydrolysis of plasma membrane lipids to form inositol triphosphate and diacylglycerol.
    B. prompts increased Ca^{++} entry into the cell from the extracellular space.
    C. causes release of bound calcium from the sarcoplasmic reticulum.
    D. elevates cytosolic Ca^{++} concentrations.
    E. probably causes all of the above.

71. Elevation of the cytosolic Ca^{++} concentration above 10^{-6} M
    A. activates phosphatase conversion of myosin phosphate into myosin.
    B. frees calmodulin for binding to actin.
    C. leads to vascular muscle cell contraction involving the interaction of actin and myosin.
    D. inactivates myosin kinase.
    E. causes all of the above.

72. All of the following naturally occurring substances are vasodilator agents *except*
    A. calcitonin gene-related peptide (CGRP).
    B. VIP.
    C. ACh.
    D. nitric oxide.
    E. Ca^{++}.

73. All of the following naturally occurring substances are vasoconstrictor agents *except*
    A. norepinephrine (α-adrenergic receptor stimulation).
    B. angiotensin II.
    C. bradykinin.
    D. vasopressin.
    E. leukotrienes.

74. Factors that contribute to gut mucosal cell death in nonocclusive intestinal ischemia include
    A. increased cardiac output and mesenteric vasodilation.
    B. parasympathetic stimulation and release of CGRP.
    C. digitalis and angiotensin II release.
    D. failure of oxygen countercurrent exchange to develop in the villi.
    E. stability of lysosomal membranes.

Matching

A. Gastrin
B. CCK
C. Somatostatin
D. Secretin
E. VIP
F. Histamine

75. Inhibits gastrin release when antrum is acidified

76. Inhibits parietal cell secretion of acid when antrum is acidified

77. Stimulates growth of gastric mucosa

78. Released by gastrin and acts as a paracrine to stimulate acid secretion

79. Stimulates gallbladder contraction in response to fat in the duodenum

80. Stimulates intestinal secretion and relaxes smooth muscle

ANSWERS

1. A		41. B	
2. D		42. E	
3. C		43. B	
4. A		44. D	
5. A		45. E	
6. C		46. B	
7. B		47. E	
8. A		48. A	
9. D		49. E	
10. B		50. D	
11. A		51. C	
12. C		52. B	
13. D		53. C	
14. C		54. D	
15. B		55. A	
16. E		56. C	
17. C		57. D	
18. C		58. A	
19. D		59. A	
20. E		60. E	
21. D		61. B	
22. B		62. B	
23. C		63. A	
24. D		64. C	
25. C		65. D	
26. B		66. C	
27. E		67. B	
28. E		68. D	
29. E		69. A	
30. C		70. E	
31. D		71. C	
32. A		72. E	
33. C		73. C	
34. B		74. C	
35. A		75. C	
36. D		76. C	
37. C		77. A	
38. B		78. F	
39. E		79. B	
40. A		80. E	

Index

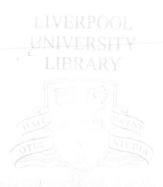